REMEDIES FOR SORROW

TO MY MOM

who taught me how to love

"*Before you know kindness as the deepest thing inside,
you must know sorrow as the other deepest thing.*"

—NAOMI SHIHAB NYE

CONTENTS

PROLOGUE

I have a photograph I've looked at more than any others. It's a picture of my two oldest children on the day my second daughter was born. Zaley, our toddler, is embracing our newborn, Anna, on a bed. Their lower halves are wrapped in a knit, off-white blanket; Zaley is wearing a heather gray romper, and Anna's upper body is bare. Anna is looking toward the window, as if she sees something no one else does. One errant chunk of her hair is angled upward, as though in good humor or resistance to the neutral-colored background of perfection I'd prepared. You can't tell they're in a hospital except for the plastic identification bracelet clipped around Anna's tiny wrist, which bears no diagnosis, just her name and her weight.

An in-house hospital photographer had taken this picture as part of a set—an invaluable gift from my parents after Anna's birth. For years, I looked at it closely, asking myself, What had I missed? Was there some sign in her searching eyes or the pallor of her skin that might have indicated she was sick? Was there a clue in the way Anna was looking, as my mom put it, "almost wistfully" toward the sun?

Now I know that there were no clues, no outward symptoms—as we tend to expect of infectious diseases—and this is the key to understanding what she has. What I sought cannot be found in those images because the story is underneath them, deeper than her skin, millions of years old, and buried by factors physical, historical, and cultural that continue to layer themselves, blanket-like, over one of the most dangerous—but overlooked—diseases in the world.

Now I also know I was asking the wrong question. I hadn't missed anything. I had felt Anna's differences from the very beginning. But because of the complex love and sorrow of motherhood, because of the silences that others expect of mothers, I doubted myself.

The question I now ask when I look at that picture is much bigger than me. The question is: *Why is the field of medicine still dismissing my daughter's disease?*

I've found many answers over the course of the last seven years.

But I've also found something else.

———

I don't remember who first told me about Saint Thomas Aquinas's "Remedies for Sorrow." I think I disregarded the idea initially, not being drawn to self-help methods—and honestly, I find his writing difficult to read. But when I applied Aquinas's remedies to the years following Anna's birth, I was surprised to find that I'd experienced his antidotes in my passage through grief. And identifying them comforted me retrospectively, proving I hadn't failed as much as I believed.

I could see that despite my husband's and my assumptions and mistakes, we had also provided healing to ourselves and our children all along by living a deeply felt, thoroughly introspected life. And if I could now voice all the silences, both medical and personal, and reveal all the treatments, both physical and spiritual, then this story might help others.

It might even prevent an entire condition.

PART I

WEEPING

"A hurtful thing hurts yet more if we keep it shut up, because the soul is more intent on it: whereas if it be allowed to escape, the soul's intention is dispersed as it were on outward things, so that the inward sorrow is lessened."

SAINT THOMAS AQUINAS

I

It's dawn when I first hear Anna's silence. The midwife is holding up my daughter, the cord between us not yet severed. She's fully formed but remarkably small, dangling in the first amber light of the sun. The tower of the hospital chapel is sounding out the tones of the half-past-five bell. My baby remains soundless, suspended—but she's alive, I can tell. She's looking at me intensely. She is black-haired and black-eyed. I know her name already.

My husband isn't there. The midwife motions for my mom to cut the cord. My mom takes scissors to the bluish rope, then places my child in my outstretched arms. For a few seconds, I'm allowed to hold her to my chest, where I can feel the deep, repeating throb of a mallet hitting a gong. Then a doctor is called. Someone slips Anna from my hands. She's brought to the corner where people huddle over her. Towels jostle her form.

"Is she okay?" I ask, again and again. Then, like a pierced bubble, her scream breaks free and fills the room.

"She's okay," the doctor or the midwife says. "But she's only five pounds."

The space changes due to her sound. The pace quickens, the shades grind up into their rectangular sockets, and now the light is a raw, painful white. A nurse demands I eat a package of graham crackers and cheese. I've had no drugs for Anna's birth, and the intensity of it is still strobe-lighting the room. I do as I'm told. Then I'm helped to a wheelchair in my nightgown, which is bright red with purple satin trim. I look a little more regal than I'd planned for an event that has destroyed me like this.

The nurse brings Anna to me, swaddled. Her hat is too big, with tiny stripes and an oversize bow. My mom appears, holding out my phone, and says, "You need to call Luke."

My husband is asleep on the fog-embalmed island in southeast Alaska where he fishes for salmon from May to September. It's three a.m. there. But he answers.

"I'm holding our baby," I tell him.

"You are?" he responds, the sleep still like gravel in his voice. "Is everything okay?"

"Yes," I say, "but she's small."

"I'll take the first flight tonight," he replies.

Anna is quiet. Her eyes, on mine, are shiny. The nurse rolls us out of the room and into an empty tiled hallway.

"Hear that?" she says. "They're playing that song for your baby, for her birthday."

The song is Brahms's "Lullaby." The beauty of the violin is a blade, cleaving me to pieces. I'm so proud, I can barely breathe.

The recovery room faces west. When the pain recedes enough, I leave the bed. I sit in a rocking chair by the window and look alternately at the bruise-colored line of the Rocky Mountains against the sky and Anna's brand-new moon-white skin. Her head is the size of a grapefruit, still wet. Her hair is matted down in tiny dark swirls. And her eyes, in this light, are magnificently deep and huge, with tentative rays of gray reaching from her pupils into an oceanic blue. During those first newborn hours when babies can be spacey and sleepy, Anna stays awake. There's something different, even foreign, about this child, like she might contain something that isn't quite ours.

Luke calls again. He's on his boat now, squeezing in one last day of fishing so we can afford for him to come home. I can picture him in his orange fishing overalls, the white sky, his silver boat, the rolling black sea. Mountains in every direction, like they might be able to stop the colossal heaving of the ocean.

We'd planned it this way months earlier—for Luke to be in Alaska and me to be in Denver—knowing he would miss Anna's birth. I'd had an unexpected C-section with Zaley, my firstborn, and the recovery had nearly undone me—the feeling of swollen ropes in my abdomen, the painfulness of laughter, the inability to walk around the block for nearly two months. For my second, I wanted a chance at a nonsurgical labor.

The OB in Sitka had said no, when I'd called from Colorado, still pregnant with Anna. I could not try for a vaginal birth, he said, even though I pointed out that it posed the same risk for me, statistically, as any woman having her first child. It seemed I understood my risk better than the doctor. And yet I would be the one held accountable for endangering my baby. He would be happy to schedule my second cesarean.

For the first and only time in my life, I preferred Luke's absence: I couldn't have this baby in Sitka, where he'd be fishing seven days a week, and I'd be recovering from an operation on a remote island with a nursing newborn and a toddler whose favorite phrase was *I want to do something!* And while it would have been illegal to force a laboring woman into surgery, I took the OB in Sitka seriously. I respect doctors, I tend to be obedient to authority, and I didn't yet think of motherhood as an authority of its own.

Over the phone, I can hear the clang of Luke's rods going into their stands, the beep of his radio when he powers it down.

"Her name is Anna," I tell him. "Anna Ruth."

Anna means "full of grace." And it's June 19—my grandma Ruth's hundredth birthday. My dad is in Chicago for her birthday party.

There's a pause as Luke's calm, deep voice covers the country between us, and then he says, "That's perfect."

Everything's perfect except for the feeling that everything isn't.

———

Since the 1960s, the public health department in every U.S. state has required that newborn babies, within the first few days of birth, be tested for a battery of diseases and disorders through their blood, which a nurse extracts from the infant's heel with a tiny stapler-type tool. Those first bulbs of blood are then stamped on an index-size card and compose the Newborn Dried Blood Spot, commonly referred to in medicine as the DBS. Once the baby's heel has yielded enough blood for five hole-punch-size circles, the card is transported to a lab, where the presence of thirty-some childhood illnesses is assayed. Diseases like phenylketonuria, maple syrup urine disease, cystic fibrosis, and sickle cell anemia are identified by the test, their names already a part of the medical canon, no matter how few or how many children they affect.

When Zaley was born in 2012, I was not prepared for this taking of her blood. I didn't expect to see her bleed until she was older—a child mobile enough to fall. The DBS doesn't require a parent's written consent, and no one offered to explain it, either. This conversation is absent for nearly every woman holding her newborn child. When I offered Zaley's heel to be punctured, it was the first time I wondered if my lack of knowledge implicated me in my daughter's pain.

Holding Anna now, I realize I'd forgotten to look up the test and its diseases. I ready Anna's bone-colored foot. I love this appendage to a ridiculous extent already, the sheen of her pearly heel, her raisin-size big toe.

A nurse pops it with the blade. Anna screams. Not enough blood comes out—her veins are too small. The nurse squeezes again till the foot is a furious purpled web. Then on the underside, the blood appears, pinprick small, and the nurse presses it down on the card. The nurse leaves with the newborn test, and I never see her again.

I never see the blood on the card again, either. When I picture it today, it's in a landfill or a dark hospital basement, nearly turned to dust, even though the specimen might hold a clue to the unexplained disabilities of millions of children around the world.

The rotating doctors arrive next, and they seem weird. They always come in sets of two. They're pediatricians from Children's Hospital, they say, and they congratulate me, but their tone is noncongratulatory. They carry clipboards, poised. One takes Anna to the plastic-walled bassinet, which is near the window. (I am so instinctively protective of her body, I won't place her in it at all after her birth.) One of the doctors indents Anna's abdomen, the other one frowns. They don't offer the possibility of disease.

I'm sitting up, chipper—*So? Everything okay?*—believing that the perkier and less emotional I seem, the better care I will receive. But they just look up like they're surprised to see me, then one smiles tightly and nods and says, "She's a beautiful baby."

She is, but she's also more than that, I can sense. I just don't know what question to ask. When they leave, they sound like shoes, and the door latch clicks with finality. They won't have answers. They might not come back. I'm hungry.

I order room service like a queen: fat, mayonnaise-filled sandwiches with fries on the side. Vanilla pudding and redundant Jell-O that jiggles happily when an aproned lady rolls the tray into my room. Anna has no rash, no seizures, no outward trouble breathing. There's no red flag, except the one inside my sternum, which feels like a damp fabric, flapping wildly, unseen.

A nurse comes in and washes Anna's ink-black hair over the sink. When she hands my child back to me, her head smells warm, like sugar cookies and soap. But her eyes are sharp, boring into me in a language I don't yet know.

———

In the late afternoon, a young woman rolls the second requirement of the newborn screening program into the room: The hearing test cart contains a baby-holding tray and a computer with wires sticking out of it that will go inside Anna's ears. These electric earbuds will emit loud clicks, prompting an instinctual response in Anna's innermost ear if she can hear sound.

Up until the 1990s, most children didn't have their hearing checked in the hospital ; deafness often went undetected till the age of three or four, permanently altering the way a child's brain could form and communicate complex thoughts. But when Anna is born, in 2015, 98 percent of American infants will have their hearing tested before they're discharged since hearing loss is the most common abnormality in infants from birth—and frequently a sign of systemic disease. Unbeknownst to me, the unassuming metal cart in the room is evidence of something I will strive for during the rest of Anna's early childhood: proven research leading to major policy changes in pediatric public health.

The hearing technician inserts the wires into Anna's ears and tells me the test will be quick. I remember the test from Zaley's first days.

But this time I know Anna will fail. It's as clear to me as the fact that labor produces a child.

The woman puts her hand on Anna's chest to steady her as she starts the test. I hold my breath, trying to create an even deeper silence than the one that exists. I can hear the muffled clicks and see that Anna is falling asleep through them. After a few minutes, the technician pulls the cords from Anna's ears. Then she gently swaddles Anna while I wait, almost out of air. Only when Anna touches my hands does she say, "I'm sorry, but she actually failed on both sides."

Anna is looking at me. I have nothing to give her, no explanation, no voice.

The hearing technician says she will retest the next day, and if Anna doesn't pass that one, I need to have her tested again in a week. She gives me no hope that Anna will be able to hear—which I appreciate later—just the information the wires have given her: sound met with silence. The technician leaves, and Anna and I lie in heavy quiet, the bale of my anxiety like weighted oxygen all around us.

In Susan Sontag's *Illness as Metaphor,* she writes: "Everyone who is born holds dual citizenship, in the kingdom of the well and in the kingdom of the sick. Although we all prefer to use only the good passport, sooner or later each of us is obliged, at least for a spell, to identify ourselves as citizens of that other place." Before having Anna, I conceived of health and sickness as Sontag presents them: two territories, the second of which I would reach on my own two feet—through old age, or an unexpected diagnosis that would be mine alone to bear. But in those first hours of Anna's life, her silence beckons me to a third place: the border between health and sickness where we will live together.

This feels like foreign soil. The American prenatal system did not prepare me, as an expecting mother, for the possibility of a disabling contagion. My OBs and midwives had implied that genetic testing and a healthy lifestyle were the best practices of pregnancy, that the twenty-week anatomy scan would reveal any complications, and that the list of disorders in their paperwork was comprehensive, would leave no large stone unturned.

Luke and I were healthy, we had no history of medical conditions in our families, and it was the fall of 2014: we were—as yet—a country largely unbothered by the risk of grave infectious disease. Viruses that threatened all of humanity were a thing of the past, I'd thought, and if they leaked through our borders, it was in small, combatable numbers, as with fleeting outbreaks of measles, Ebola, TB—fairly nonthreatening flare-ups, quickly squelched by a trustworthy (but vague) public health system designed to prevent and protect.

As for epidemics in American *children,* those belonged more to the realm of fiction than to real, current-day life. These kinds of plagues happened only prevaccines, in the pioneer literature I had read as a child and would later read to my kids: malaria in *Little House on the Prairie*, scarlet fever in *Little Women*—both diseases so rampant as to be expected, and that presented with symptoms the parents could see.

No, an infectious disease simply does not occur to me while I'm considering Anna's anomalies; she has only lived inside me, where things had been handled appropriately. Like any well-read woman in the twenty-first century, I'd understood the fundamentals of pregnancy: no kitty litter (it can carry toxoplasmosis), alcohol (which can cause fetal alcohol syndrome), lunch meats (which carry listeria, very rarely), or sushi (due to high levels of mercury). Aside from these standard no-no's, I figured if I needed to worry about something contagious and dangerous to her gestation, then my doctors, the CDC, and the internet would have warned me.

I assumed I was protected from the illnesses of others by my location, my education level, and the American healthcare system. And with Anna in utero, there had been no threatening elsewhere or others: Alaska and Colorado, Luke and me, and our daughter and her friends.

Never, at any of my twenty-some prenatal appointments, had I been told that in the combination above, there was a serious risk.

In 1975 the journalist Nicholas von Hoffman put it like this: "The idea of preventive medicine is faintly un-American. It means, first, recognizing that the enemy is us."

❖

Anna nurses well, I watch her sleep. When she wakes up, I look at her, and she looks at me. To increase her blood sugar levels, I do the only thing I've been instructed to do: I wrap us up, skin to skin, inside a hospital-sheet cocoon.

But when the doctors come on their rounds again and note her failed hearing test with a light scratch of pen on paper, the alarm inside me rings. When I ask if her failed test and being small for gestational age (SGA) are connected, I'm prodding them to identify something that causes both. But they don't. They explain them as coincidental events—she probably has fluid stuck in her ears because she's petite; she'll probably pass the test when her ears grow and it drains.

It seems the doctors know best, and yet ironically, I'm left to solve the mystery myself. My midwife pops by, congratulates me on the natural birth, and says we can leave the next morning.

That afternoon my mom brings Zaley to meet the baby. Zaley has a creamy blond bowl cut that shimmies above a body in perpetual motion. She talks in complex sentences, somersaults spontaneously, can recite every type of Pacific salmon. We'd assumed our next child would be just as ambitious, would arrive early at gross motor milestones, babbling, then speech. But Anna's presence has already inverted our relationship to speed.

My mom's footsteps stop outside the doorway. And under the privacy curtain, I can see Zaley's size-five feet stalled in place, too, clad in white folded socks and her favorite dirt-caked tennies. Zaley has never approached anything so slowly. She's just begun her (lifelong) phase of choosing her outfits for herself, and when she emerges in a fancy and layered tea-length gown, she pauses after one step, barely inside the room. Her hands are holding each other, her eyes wide on the baby—this thing we'd discussed, who's now a person, who is here.

"Come here, sweetie," I say, remembering the overpowering

panic of love when I first saw her. But even when beckoned, Zaley hesitates with uncharacteristic reserve.

A few seconds later she tiptoes over, clambers up the side of the bed, and settles at my side. Without a sound, she takes in Anna's miniature size, her otter-black hair, the sheer fact that this is her sister.

"Annaroof," Zaley whispers, all one word, cupping one hand gently over the top of the baby's head. Then she looks up at me and asks, "Is she okay?"

I have seen Zaley with other infants, and this is different. It's a worry that has no reason, just a presence. It's like she, too, senses something bigger than we've encountered before.

"I don't know," I say back.

That first and final evening in the hospital, Luke's parents come to meet the baby, and then our priest, his wife, and Anna's godparents arrive to sing the Russian Orthodox prayers of birth over her. I don't tell these close friends about the failed tests. It feels like I'll be telling a secret only Anna and I know. I listen to the familiar rise and fall of the Byzantine tones, the songs Luke had sung throughout my pregnancy, his voice the sound of all my askings. We anoint Anna with oil, drawing inch-size, scented crosses on her head, her hands, her eyes, her ears.

Later, when we know what Anna has, we begin to pray for miracles.

Really, Anna's first miracle is that she was born at all.

2

The air is warm and close the next morning, as if I've been bound in gauze. Anna is asleep next to me on the bed when I hear the door creak open, then the quiet of a person trying to be quiet, and there stands Luke. He has slept on the floor of the Seattle airport and taken the six a.m. His cheeks are pink from fishing, and I can tell he's gained a few pounds from eating Pizza Express frequently over the last six weeks. Looking at him after our seasonal separations sends a hot zing through me—his thick biceps, ample lips, Coors-colored beard. He holds me tight in the doorway for a few seconds before we face the baby on the bed.

"She's so small," he whispers. "I'm afraid to touch her."

"It's fine, you get used to it," I say.

Anna is the size of a guinea pig. Luke slides one palm under her head, then one under her back, but he could hold her entirely in just one of his hook-calloused hands. His eyes go wide as though he's both afraid of her and in awe of her, and I remember the way he first looked as a father—sturdy, scared, tender in his everyday Carhartts.

"She failed her second hearing test when you were traveling," I tell him.

"We don't know anything yet," he says, not looking up, in love already.

I want to leave the hospital: the beeping and the fussing, the clinical feel that something might go wrong at any moment. I shower quickly, and my dark curls drip down the back of a long black nursing dress. We're having Anna's "shotgun" baptism that day, Anna's second day, before Luke will turn around in forty-eight hours and leave for Alaska again. My mom and I have planned to fly to Alaska with the girls ten days after that.

A nurse offers me Vicodin and a wheelchair, but I refuse and ask for a few Tylenol instead. Another hospital worker shows us the padding he's added to Anna's car seat for infants born premature, even though Anna was born full term. We've filled out her birth certificate paperwork, she has eaten and peed, and our discharge is complete, even though it feels like we're illegally taking Anna from a place she still needs to be. In the hallway, Luke says, "Hang on, I forgot something important," and darts back into the room. He emerges with two giant nursing jugs—thirty-two-ounce water bottles that have a handle, an accordion straw, and a picture of a bare-shouldered woman gazing down at her newborn child. Luke likes to use these in public, with no shame, in the months after I give birth.

Better equipped for hydration, at least, we lumber carefully down the stairs, my husband, my fragile child, and I. But the stairs feel like they're barely there. All former stability has undergone a silent but seismic shift.

Past the sliding hospital doors, the sun feels relentless and harsh. I canopy my eyes with one hand as Luke fetches his truck, and in this blinding exposure, I long deeply for Alaska, for its shield of precipitation and its abundance of grays—which surprises me because every year, I viscerally dread going back. Instead of riding up front when Luke pulls up, I squeeze into the back next to Anna, my vigilance beginning.

Before Anna was born, when we'd hatched our plans to bring a newborn across the country, we always tacked on the statement *as long as she's healthy, of course*, as though saying it meant she would be (and that it was the only thing that mattered). Now reality is dripping in: What if she isn't healthy? If she's sick, has God allowed this illness? And will we be able to provide for her needs in Alaska, whatever they might be?

Luke looks at me in the rearview mirror and asks if I'm okay, and I say yes, even though my nipples are already cracked and bleeding and slathered with clear jelly under my dress. I don't talk about how I feel like an overfull cup with my emotions sloshing over every edge. I don't voice the feral anxiety that is scraping up my throat. I could tell Luke, but I don't want to worry him when he has the pressure of Alaska and leaving us alone. The reality of the postpartum period seems to belong in a box labeled with the same phrase I'll later find implied about Anna's disease: *Better left unsaid*.

Luke reaches back, and I hold one of his hands and one of Anna's the whole way to St. Elizabeth's, our church.

———

Eight years prior, on a snowy Sunday afternoon, I'd met Luke for the first time at St. Elizabeth's. My oldest brother, David, was in Catholic seminary at the time and had suggested I come see a Byzantine church—one of several smaller Eastern Catholic churches shadowed by the Roman Catholic church and nearly identical, liturgically, to Russian Orthodoxy. Reluctant to attend, I'd been unexpectedly moved by the rich sensory details of the space. Under a vanilla-colored dome, hand-painted icons stood on narrow, gilded stands. Parishioners didn't sit; they walked, bowed down, gently kissed the paintings of the saints. A thin plume of incense ribboned into the room, catching the sun as it swirled. Something there seemed more palpable to me than it had in all my Sundays growing up: perhaps there was something invokable and knowable around us, even if it was something we couldn't fully understand.

There was no cry room; children roamed freely and loudly around the church—at one point, sweeping their hands against the priest's robe, to impart healing, as he passed. (Some of these children were the priest's kids, I would later learn; Orthodox and Eastern Catholic priests can marry before they're ordained.) Different from the Roman Catholic church in which I'd been raised, something here felt authentic, ancient, laid bare.

What struck me most, though, was what I heard: no instruments, just melody and harmony curling around each other, midair. It was tear-inducing, prickling my skin—then it all swooped down to silence and goose-bumped me again. There were six or seven choir members. And one of them was the most attractive guy I had ever seen.

Luke was wearing a navy blue sweater and jeans, and his voice— the tenor line—seemed to lift above the others and hover there in the smoky shafts of light. I tried not to look at him, but I could hear him even without looking, and I knew (alongside a little prayer that went *Please God, let him not be gay, married, or in seminary*) that he was it for me.

After church, the people gathered for a potluck in a space with skinny, sun-filled windows, and I watched the choirboy set up chairs and then pour coffee for everyone in the room. When he finally sat down across from me, he said, "I'm Luke," simple, unwavering. He looked at me for longer than a person usually looks at a person. Good thing I married him, or I would have thought about him for the rest of my life.

Luke was the oldest of six boys, he said, and when I asked what he did for a living, he mentioned—in his characteristic downplaying way—that he had a small salmon-guiding business in Sitka, Alaska, during the summer. Most people associate Sitka, Alaska, with the Sitka in the Sandra Bullock rom-com *The Proposal*, which features stony mountains, affluent homes, and cedar forests, all filmed . . . on the coast of Maine. That movie hadn't come out yet, but I definitely conjured something more Hollywood-Alaska than what Sitka really is. And I know I asked Luke what the elevation of Sitka was—a town where he *fished*. On the *sea*.

I was nervous, Luke is easygoing. I was teaching high school English at the time, in New Orleans actually, and I was just home for a few weeks. But I saw May in front of me as clear as day: I would wrap up finals, book a ticket, and see what Luke's life was like.

Every time Luke visited me, for the rest of that spring, I would ask him to sing. When I thought of him, I thought of the sound of him first—his deep and confident voice over the phone; his mouth, in that church, sending up the Psalms. From the very beginning, our relationship was built on the foundation of sound.

———

Though my prenatal care providers hadn't prepared me for illness, my religion should have. In scripture, God is referred to constantly as a healer; in Orthodoxy, as the Great Physician. Meaning, then, that we are all vectors of sickness, whether inherent or acquired, physical or mental. According to Orthodox teaching, this does not mean we are culpable or less worthy of love; it means we need more than ourselves. This I feel sharply after Anna's birth.

Climbing the steps to the church, I regret not accepting the pain-killer from the nurse. The church has no air conditioning, and my vagina feels like it might drop out of my body like a part coming loose from a car. Luke joins the choir in the corner, and the girls and I slide into a pew in front of Luke's parents and mine. Anna is wearing the cream-colored gown Luke wore as a child. When the prayers begin, they have more allusions to sickness and healing than I'd been aware of before. "That this water may prove effectual for the averting of every plot of visible and invisible enemies," Father Chrysostom prays over the font where Anna will be submerged. "Make it a fountain of incorruption, a gift of sanctification, a loosing of sins, a healing of sicknesses."

I have always loved the elevated diction of the Orthodox liturgy, but now it's like I'd never really listened with motive or precision. For a second, I wonder if Anna can hear the words, too, but I remember what the doctors said—that it's just fluid in her ears, that it will pass—and I adopt this belief, cling to it, reject any notion she might be deaf.

At one point during the service, the priest lays the baby on the ground, and the mother comes and picks the child up. It has always moved me, this gesture of isolation met by rescue, and when I hinge down in my pained body and lift Anna from the floor, I can sense that my responsibility to her will be greater than I understand.

After church, we have a party in the same room where I first spoke to Luke. It's lit by the same tall windows and silvery-blue wallpaper that has always been there. It's full of the long white tables Luke has always set up and taken down. Like all the other baptisms we've had in our community, there is vodka being poured and people singing "Many Years" and a huge cake being cut into squares. But now there's this snow-colored baby, asleep again, draped over Luke's back, and looking at her throws a blanket of unfamiliarity over the room.

———

Two days later Luke leaves for Alaska. His absence is a chasm, no matter how planned his departures. I take Anna to the hospital again, where she fails another hearing test. And this time I cry from a place much more muscular than my eyes. The nurse places her hand on my shoulder, and my sobs are shaking her arm. From far away, she says we should see an audiologist—if they'll see us on such short notice—before we leave for Alaska. Do I want her to make some calls? I nod. She calls four, finds one. It's not close, but they'll see us the next day.

———

At home, I nurse and pump, nurse and pump. When I'm done being sucked, I let Zaley play with the breast pump knobs. She's an airplane pilot, heading to Sitka, Alaska. She needs copious lactation cookies to stay focused for the duration of the flight. I pretend to ignore the roar of my anxiety, but when that game is over, I let Zaley watch *Mary Poppins* because it's two and a half hours long.

The next morning I take Zaley to my mom's, and from there I drive on a fast highway to a modern-looking hospital where I will find out, yet again, whether my baby is hearing. The audiologist is young, and I resent how long it looks like she was able to spend getting ready in the morning. She sticks electrodes all over Anna's head and tells me to hold her as still as I can *for the next two hours*. While Anna providentially obeys, the auditory brainstem response (ABR) measures her brain wave activity in response to sound.

At the end of the test, the audiologist tells me quietly that Anna's brain didn't respond to sounds at all.

While I sit stunned, the audiologist says it's still early, Anna is still small, and we should have more testing done in a month. I hold the back of my hand up to my mouth and cry as quietly as I can, as though emitting sound would be a betrayal of the way Anna is.

"One last thing," the audiologist says. "Is there any genetic hearing loss in either of your families?"

"Not that I know of," I answer.

She does not mention that there's one infectious disease that causes more hearing loss and deafness in children all over the world than any other nongenetic cause.

———

In the audiology community, providers strive for a model commonly known as the "1-3-6" approach to treatment: the baby will have their hearing tested before one month of age; they will be diagnosed by three months of age; and they will receive intervention by six months of age. *Intervention* means education for the baby so they can reach their potential, whether that's becoming fluent in sign language or speech, or only being able to express their most basic needs. In the United States, the first goal is close to being met. The second goal is not: over 60 percent of children who fail their hearing screening never receive a documented diagnosis. And less than half are enrolled in early intervention services before they're six months old.

———

Back at home, Anna's phantom diagnosis follows me through our house, while I pack raincoats for Alaska, carry my soundless baby from room to room, and try to occupy a toddler who wants to paint and run a lemonade stand and aggressively snuggle the baby anytime I put her down. Gone is the alternate universe of the hospital and its quiet remove, and here is the painful reality of two young children and my husband at a great distance. Zaley wants to be in Alaska NOW. Or she wants to go swimming at six in the morning—my favorite thing to do with her, and a loss I didn't anticipate before having a second child. Anna never reacts to any of Zaley's impassioned requests, and her oblivious quiet imposes on me a volume of its own.

I know maybe I shouldn't go to Alaska, but the fear of doing everything without Luke is unthinkable. I'm doing that now, and it feels like a withering.

———

Luke's mom, Anita, comes over. The seventh child in a line of towering brunettes, Anita is of average height, very slender, and has short blond hair. She's always impeccably dressed, and she tells it like it is. After raising six boys and tending to the messes that came with them, her attention to detail is beyond impressive. She's slipping Anna into a clean onesie when she notes that her right arm is less elastic than her left. Lifting one arm, then the other, over Anna's head, she shows me that the right arm won't pull straight. Anita had a child who was different, too: her sixth boy, Max, was born with craniosynostosis—a malformation where his skull lacked a soft spot at birth, necessitating a surgery, while he was an infant, to have part of his cranium removed. His seizures came next.

I can feel the heat and sting that precede tears when I tell Anita I feel like something bigger, something as yet unmentioned, is wrong. Anna no longer wants to nurse on the right, turn her head to the right, or unclench her right fist, which is never relaxed. She never sleeps for more than a minute in the car because the Moro reflex (the *oh-crap* one, where the baby's arms fly up like they're falling through space) kicks in as soon as she enters sleep.

Anita cups her hands behind Anna's head and beholds her, undistracted, as if Anna were the most valuable trophy a person could win. But she doesn't discredit my concerns. She knew something was up with Max in utero, before any doctors did. She knows that when mothers sense a veil over their child, they're the first to lift the edge, to peer under the protective covering.

Some friends—maybe out of fear or maybe out of hopefulness, but likely out of both—prefer to insist on the health they've already imagined into the body of my daughter. It's not in our nature to embrace the atypical or to allow illness, at least initially, the possibility of power. "Don't worry, she'll catch up!" they say when they bring dinner. Or "Did you see that? She turned toward your voice!" But I know differently. This is a feeling untouched by the false reassurance most of us are so keen on giving. It's clear only to me: she isn't hearing. It's clear only to me: we're missing something we can't yet see.

3

My whole adult life I have protected myself with silence in medical situations. At the risk of seeming weak, abrasive, hysteric, obsessive, or pushy, I don't ask all the questions I have of any medical professional I see. Which is why, when I get to the pediatrician's office and a smiling nurse leads me to a lamplit room with an oatmeal-colored couch where I can nurse my ten-day-old before weighing her on the scale, I don't ask the nurse to turn the emo music off, even though it must be grating on any postpartum mom. I place Anna on my huge left boob—the only side she'll take from now on—knowing it won't suffice. And I practice the quiet I've learned to adopt.

After all, the last time I voiced my concerns, during my pregnancy with Anna, I'd basically been refused entry from the clinic that was supposed to take care of me. Early in my second trimester, I'd had a severe, persistent cold that felt like mono, and after I left a message for my OB, the nurse had called me back and said: "If you're that sick, you shouldn't come in."

Who knows—maybe my OB believed my complaints to be somatization: not physical illness but questionable self-reported symptoms arising from emotional distress. That characterization is attributed overwhelmingly to women, even when they do have a discernible disease. In the United States, women in the middle of a heart attack are seven times more likely to be sent home from the hospital than men. And this glaring disparity shows up in medical research as well: of the $42 billion the National Institutes of Health spend on medical research each year, only $5 billion is specifically allocated to issues in women's health.

So even in Dr. Kono's office where I've always felt seen and heard,

I feel the American medical system's legacy of pinning women's problems on hysteria and hormones, not on valid concerns. No, I won't mention the sadness streaming into the room through the speakers. Because if my child, for some reason, has contracted something that began inside me, during pregnancy, that means it's a woman's disease. And that means I need to be cool and collected to earn a diagnosis.

And that is what I'm here to obtain.

Silently, I'm also anxious as hell because we're leaving for Alaska the next day, and I'd like the pediatrician's permission before we leave. From the couch where Anna is too-slowly drinking, I look at the pictures of children they have on the walls: hearing, standing, smiling, seeing—no hearing aids, walkers, wheelchairs, or glasses. These pictures wound me now, even though I've been looking at them for years. As soon as your life changes, you see everything differently—even what's not there.

I meet the nurse in the hallway, as instructed, with Anna's warm back in the palms of my hands. The nurse weighs her, and I watch, in shock, when the first number doesn't tick upward beyond a four. The nurse says, "She's a little one, isn't she?" and directs us back to the couch. Then Dr. Kono comes in.

A writer himself, he published a book of poetry during his residency about his time caring for severely ill children, children who would never become adults. Dr. Kono has seen Zaley for years, he knows about our lives in Alaska, and he's easy for me to trust. He's a young father and Stanford-educated, with round black glasses, dark skin, and a slight frame, and he doesn't do the song-and-dance routine our pediatric dentist does that makes me embarrassed for her.

I can't handle anything but honesty at this point, and honesty is all I have to give. Just that morning, while driving to the doctor's office, I felt like I might have a little freak-out. I wasn't sure what that was going to look like, but I pictured a plate shattering and my hair going all crazy, and I was saying the Jesus Prayer on repeat: *Lord Jesus Christ, have mercy on me.* For days, Luke has been asking me over the phone if I'm okay, and all I can say is no. I'm mad that he's gone, even though I know he has to be. I'm mad that even though I consider myself independent, his distance increases the gravity of all our problems.

Dr. Kono sits down on the stool, folds his hands. We go through the basic newborn checklist, and then he asks me the same thing every hearing technician and doctor has asked me so far: "Is she startling to any sounds?" No, I tell him, no, not ever. This always feels like the incorrect answer.

"Can I hold her?" Dr. Kono asks, holding out his hands—a warm consolation, as opposed to the cold, papered table. "Hmm. She is small," he says, orienting her face up on his lap. "She also failed her hearing tests?" I nod. He doesn't say more. He presses his hands gently into her lungs. He brings her feet in toward her hips, then back out, like a little unaffected frog. He looks in her eyes and her ears, rubs small circles on her neck. Every motion he performs, though gentle, is like clicking a ratchet strap tighter and tighter around my core. Just when I think I can't take a breath, he hands her back to me and rolls his stool away.

"She seems pretty healthy," he says, fingers folded again. "But if you have time today, I want to test her for a little-known virus that can cause hearing loss and smallness at birth. It's called congenital CMV."

"What if she has it?" I ask. It's the first time I've heard the letters *CMV*. I figure maybe it's something like the flu, and it will go away within a week.

"CMV is a common virus that stays in your system forever, like chicken pox," he says. "If you caught it when you were pregnant, it wouldn't harm you. But if it crosses the placenta, it can pose serious problems for a fetus because they're in the midst of development."

"If she has it," I ask, flinching, "can you treat her for it?"

"There's an aggressive treatment for newborns. In some cases, it can reverse hearing loss and stop the progression of the virus. But you have to start the medication during the first month of life."

The word *reverse* stands out, like some kind of wizardry that might undo Anna's inabilities.

"How do you test her for it?" I ask.

"It's a simple urine catch," Dr. Kono tells me, stool stalled in place, no preparation to leave the room till I acquiesce. "The nurse will strap what she calls a 'potty purse' onto Anna, and hopefully she'll pee into it before you have to leave." He's quiet then, undisturbed by the silence, as I weigh my options.

"Do you think I can still go to Alaska tomorrow?" I ask, feeling like a child.

"I think so," he says. "We won't get the CMV results back till you're up there. But a pediatrician in Sitka can temporarily direct her care."

So I agree to the test. Susie, an older nurse with spiky blond hair and a jaguar-print sweater, comes in. We've seen her before; she's blunt and spunky, and I like her. On goes the potty purse—a transparent pouch like a miniature sandwich bag, attached with clear, easy-peel tape. I nurse Anna, and she fills the bag with a triangle of pale yellow pee. Susie folds a new diaper onto Anna with gentle finesse.

"Whatever you find out, love, it'll be okay," she says. She has adult sons with medical issues, she says, and they have shaped her life. It's my first glimpse that what we're facing might be life-altering, but I clamp down into confident denial. I smile, keeping the idea of disability where it belongs—in the anecdotes of others. I'm doing what most educated mothers might do in this situation: rationalizing that because I'd read pregnancy blogs and pregnancy memoirs and evidence-based pregnancy guides, this "common" virus couldn't really be that common, or I'd have heard of it before—therefore it can't be happening to me.

I click Anna into her car seat and pack up our things. In the hallway, I pluck a mermaid sticker off the counter to bring back home to Zaley.

———

Unless you've heard of CMV, you will not Google CMV. You will not go to the CDC's website—as I do, while Zaley is napping and Anna is looking up from my lap—and click ten circuitous links to reach the information they have posted about CMV. It's only when you're facing a diagnosis of congenital CMV (when the information is nine months too late) that you begin to learn about the disease—a condition the medical world has contested disclosing for the last seventy-some years.

The basics appear quickly, impartially at first, on the screen: CMV stands for *cytomegalovirus*, and *congenital* isn't related to congestive as I'd always assumed; congenital means "from birth." The CDC's website explains: "Over half of adults by age 40 have been infected with CMV. Most people infected with CMV show no signs or symptoms. When a baby is born with cytomegalovirus (CMV) infection, it is called congenital CMV."

Instantly, I feel calmed by the tone and content of the CDC. There's no urgency here. If CMV simply happens to the majority of adults and is seemingly unpreventable, it must not be so bad. Then I come to this fact: "By the age of five years, one in three children has been infected with CMV, but usually does not have symptoms."

I understand that these children are fine because they aren't a fragile, still-blooming fetus, as Dr. Kono had said. The problem is that toddlers have mothers. Mothers who might be trying to have their next baby and shouldn't come into contact with CMV. Next, I Google, *How long do toddlers excrete CMV?* An American Academy of Pediatrics (AAP) link appears, and I click it to read that toddlers can "shed" CMV contagiously in their saliva, urine, snot, and blood for months, even *years*.

And I had never been told.

Something happens to my eyes. It reminds me of when I'm pheasant hunting with Luke and a bird explodes from under our feet, how I black out momentarily before I see the wings rising up, desperate, into the refuge of the sky.

I have so many questions, and there are so many studies. But it only takes a few minutes to assemble the pertinent facts: if the virus is contracted by a pregnant woman through intimate contact with a CMV-infected child, it can replicate into the placenta and the uterine wall, then into the fetus, where it has the potential to impact all fetal growth. Once the baby is born, congenital CMV can manifest with visible symptoms, or the baby can look fine but exhibit *progressive* symptoms as time goes along.

And the spectrum of those symptoms is violently broad: deafness, blindness, cerebral palsy, developmental delays. Epilepsy, lung disease, autism, death. Most of which you won't be able to see at birth, all the studies make clear. And most of these symptoms will never be linked to congenital CMV without a doctor interested in looking deeper; they'll be labeled later in childhood, identified as their own separate conditions.

Gone goes the ground again, like the hospital stairs. There's a hot pounding in my now-fire-rimmed ears. If I stand up, I know the room will be cut up with holes, aswirl in black. So I sit, as though this enormous nondisclosure could be digested if I'm calm enough to allow it. I do read, with the tiniest bit of relief, that 80 percent of babies born with CMV will go on to have no symptoms at all. But then I realize that 20 percent is a large chunk, by any statistician's standards.6

And the percentages seem to silence a harrowing fact: that 100 percent of babies born with CMV have the potential to end up with permanent delays.

In concrete numbers, around 40,000 American children are born each year with CMV, of whom up to 8,000 will end up with lifelong disabilities.Children disabled by congenital CMV outnumber children disabled here by any other congenital condition or disease, including Down syndrome, spina bifida, cystic fibrosis, and pediatric HIV.

Numbers don't usually become people in our perception. But I, more than most, can intimately conceptualize CMV's reach. Sitka's population fluctuates between 6,000 and 8,000 people (depending on the size of the cruise ships docked in town), so those numbers aren't just numbers to me; they are actual human beings. They're the workers and shoppers in three grocery stores, the entire staffs of the Coast Guard base and two hospitals, the congregations at fifteen churches, the people going to the movie theater, the hikers, the artists, the trollers and long-liners and sport fishermen—every man, woman, and child on our island would be deaf, blind, disabled, and/or dead every year that we return to Sitka if I wanted to picture how many humans are annually impacted by congenital CMV, in our country alone.

I'm looking at Anna in my lap, the same baby she'll be no matter the research I unearth. But I can feel a deep churning inside me, an impulse that will both plague and direct me for as long as I live. If Anna does have CMV—which I'm still loath to believe—then her growth restriction wasn't just a random mishap during my pregnancy; this was a serious upending of her development due to a dangerous, undisclosed disease.

The last thing I read is a study from 2013, stating that congenital CMV is the leading cause of birth defects and developmental delays in the United States.

———

I'm not reading anymore; I'm watching something else that's happening on the edges of my screen. The watchful gods of the internet have been populating my laptop with ads carefully selected for pregnancy. There are Land of Nod bookshelves lining a laughably white nursery where poop must not exist; a crib that can play a recording of a mother's heartbeat and that guarantees 30 percent more sleep for the newborn at night; a photo of a pregnant woman in a wheatfield with glossy flat-iron curls, both hands on her bump, leaning down to kiss her toddler on the lips.

I don't even know what item the last picture is trying to sell—maybe an impossibly benign version of life, as advertisements do: no food smears on sweaters, no primary colors. Obviously, no existence of CMV.

I remember the me who had never been pregnant, who believed I would be like the woman above—barely weakened by childbearing or child-having, and not just in photographs but for the duration of my pregnancy and my children's early years. I was the first of my family members and friends to get pregnant, which meant I didn't have any accurate image in my head of life with very young kids. In the first weeks of pregnant thrill, I believed the lies I saw online—on social media, in pregnancy articles, in ads I passively absorbed: that pregnancy and baby-holding could be a pastoral experience if I approached it as such, through the right birth plan, wallpaper, and baby equipment. More than that, I quietly believed that through willpower and strategy, I could have a perfect pregnancy and, later, a perfect human being.

Our priest's wife—and Zaley's godmother—Marica is a therapist who has counseled a number of women expecting their first child. A mother herself to three grown boys, Marica told me once, in her graceful South African accent: "The preamble to pregnancy in America seems to be a matter of theater. People really have no idea what they're getting into."

It didn't take long, though, for me to feel shamed by the images I'd once believed could be me; by eight weeks, pregnancy for me was the opposite of serene. I was wracked by nausea and irritability and existentially terrified for the great upheaval that I knew lay in wait. I wasn't even sure when I should tell people I was pregnant, because if I miscarried, I would feel ashamed for having announced that I would imminently present a baby, and then people would see that my body had failed. I wanted to say to my audience, as the images of pregnancy had said to me: *It's going to be okay.*

Though her subject was not becoming a mother but the loss of her own, Meghan O'Rourke wrote about America today as a society that doesn't expect or embrace the ongoingness of suffering and grief. In her memoir, *The Long Goodbye,* one of her friends says to her: "There are many wonderful things about our culture, but I'm sorry, it is a phobic culture. People do not want to confront the existential mess that is life. They want to check things off—okay, you're okay."

People clearly don't want to confront the existential mess of starting life, either, if there's no honesty about this ridiculously prevalent and proximate disease called CMV. During my pregnancies, my OB had asked how many drinks I'd consumed in a week, but not how many toddlers I had in my house. I'd worried deeply about the blue cheese I'd accidentally devoured on a burger and about a bath that might have been too hot. No mention of the risk I loved most—the one who ate my food, followed me around, and sneezed into my mouth.

I'd been conditioned to fear everything and make it look like I feared nothing. Turns out, I'd spent all my anxiety and effort worrying about threats to pregnancy that occur far less often than infections with CMV.

With Anna's birth behind me and Anna's future in front of me, I see now that the biggest lie of all is a quiet and ugly one, the one I'd told myself: that if I adhered to the prescribed plan for pregnancy, then I could resemble the women I saw online. I, too, could be the glowing owner of nondisabled kids.

Today, because of advances in diagnostics and medical intervention, more pregnancies than ever are brought to term, and more infants are thriving after serious diagnoses at birth. According to the CDC, birth defects affect 1 in 33 babies born in the United States each year. Additionally, one in four adults has a disability that impacts major life activities—a number not even close to being represented by the images served to us by our media, our advertisers, or our healthcare system.

I'm sure this was partly why, as soon as Dr. Kono had explained CMV, I'd felt a reeling, recoiling *This can't be happening to me*. Even in his office, there'd been no sign of the hereness of the disabled, only an environment that depicted their absence. I had perceived disease and disability as being alarmingly nonnormative or super rare—therefore something to be deeply feared.

But now those pioneer women pop into my head. They weren't protected from any aspect of reality. They always knew the nearness of harm, illness, death. They saw the prevalence of disability in their actual population, not the diluted version of it. Those mothers were badasses because they understood, and managed, ever-present risk.

Today we don't have smallpox or malaria or polio or rubella; in most women's minds, we have all but eliminated the possibility of serious neonatal infectious disease, which is one reason our pregnancy climate is nearly unable to accommodate the discussion of congenital CMV. The other reason, I now see, looking at the ads of buxom young women practically trembling with hope, is that as technology has evolved, our advertising and social media culture has made us weaker in the face of reality, not stronger. We're desperate for the perfection that doesn't exist.

Anna has just started to cry—a mouselike, polite kind of appeal—so I close my computer. I think of Luke, who's removed from our culture by an ocean for a good chunk of the year. Right now he's probably waiting for his line to jump in some dark-watered bay, ready to accept whatever diagnosis or difference lands in our life. I, on the other hand, am shushing my sick infant with the image of every typical child burned into my brain. I'm still hoping Anna will get over what she has. I'm saying to her—to myself—the same thing O'Rourke's friend said, the same thing the doctor said right after Anna was born: *Okay, you're okay.*

As soon as I picture the CMV test in the lab, as soon as the word *positive* appears in my head, a door inside me slams.

4

As my mom, my girls, and I drive to the airport in Denver, I'm considering how the quantity of rain in Alaska dampens my quality of life. I know if Anna has major health problems *and* it pours every day, I might just dissolve. At the time, I don't realize I'm leaving out the more important considerations about bringing Anna to Sitka: the lack of a pediatric intensive care unit, the lack of access to major pharmacies, the lack of pediatric specialists.

Fortunately for me, my mom is a retired pediatric nurse who specialized in children with serious diseases—transplants, diabetes, epilepsy—though she, too, had never heard of congenital CMV. She also worked in the oncology department at Children's Hospital for five years, tending to some of the worst suffering a nurse can imagine. The flower girl in her wedding was one of her patients—a girl named Holly who wore a white bonnet to cover her hairless head. My mom says those families showed her the power of humanity over illness, even in the presence of imminent death. I'm sure it was partly the way she cared for her patients that gave them their hope. No matter what I'm going through, my mom is where I land.

She's 100 percent Irish, barely five feet tall, and prays the Rosary daily. She has short dark curls and the same blue-gray eyes as mine. She's prone to tears (unless she needs to be strong for others, and then her eyes are steely and dry), she always wears turtlenecks, and she hates to fly. The last time we flew together, in 1996, she told me, pale-faced, to use one of the flat inset phones on the seats in front of us. "Call our close relatives," she'd said in the midst of mild turbulence. "We need to say our goodbyes. This plane is going down."

So for this trip, I've forced her to double-down on the Xanax.

Which is maybe why she actually gets out of the car in the parking lot, even though one of my brothers warned me she might not. Inside, we check our bags, and more bags, and the car seats, and I do what Dr. Kono said, which is to keep Anna in a carrier, safe and away from germs. This seems a little out of order: the worst germs, if so inclined, have already had their way.

On the plane, my mom and the flight are remarkably smooth. Besides a widening of her eyes every time the plane banks sideways over the dazzle of the Pacific, my mom shows barely a sign of the anxiety I know is roiling under her skin. This veneer of calmness is something we share. No one sitting near us can fathom the depths of our distress.

Over Canada we fly, past pods of whales migrating for cooler waters and islands whose outlines have become familiar over the last decade of summers I've spent in Sitka. The woman next to my mom—also, unfortunately, afraid of flying—is my friend's oldest daughter. Three rows up, I spot two of our neighbors. This is how it is to fly to small-town Alaska. When we approach the arrowhead-shaped outline of Baranof Island, the clouds part like curtains revealing a stage, and the wing seems so close to the emerald slope of Mount Verstovia, we could jump out and land on the green. Bald eagles are gliding down the thermals in their grand and random loops, and I watch their six-foot wingspans as they tilt against a backdrop of fog rising, steamlike, from the mossy forests below.

Somewhere inside the block of anxiety that hasn't budged since Anna was born, a dormant ping of love pops up inside me for this place that is such a hardship and such a harbor in my life. Here's the lush slope where our rental home sits, our totes from the storage unit sitting inside. Here are the towering Tlingit totem poles, the Orthodox church's onion-shaped dome, the trollers and seiners and long-liners with their metal arms outstretched, unzipping the teal water below. Here's the sky-blue bridge connecting our island to the smaller island where we'll land.

"Oh, Megan," my mom says, "it's just beautiful."

Tears squeeze into the sides of my eyes. I'm proud of this half-home of ours, proud that my mom can witness this part of my life. Zaley spots a boat in the sound that looks nothing like Luke's and yells, "HEY EVERYONE, LOOK! THAT'S MY DAD!"

When I first flew to Sitka, in my twenties, my head was full of images I'd collected about Alaska online. I imagined myself as the svelte heroine of "the last frontier": kissing my hot fisherman on the dock, climbing steep mountains with friends, posing for pictures as my hair whipped artfully in arctic wind.

But when I stepped off that first flight, the mountains I'd seen in pictures were nowhere in sight. The fog was so everywhere, so soggy, it felt like it was inside my brain. And the rain was not the late-afternoon precipitation in Colorado that comes with the fanfare of fast clouds and the reward of a rainbow. Landscapes were smeared by weather, homes on the coast were drippy and shabby, glue-colored clouds emitted a cold, unpleasant spray.

Luke's friend Erik picked me up, and we drove to the seaside grocery store and purchased some warm almonds in a brown paper bag. Those nuts were the only warmth I felt or saw that day. We drove on the one main road, which skirts the coast, and Erik said, "Luke is somewhere out there," pointing at the unforgiving gray.

That first summer Luke and I lived with a married couple who didn't use heat. Their thermostat always read fifty-four degrees, and in the mornings, in a knit hat and fingerless gloves, I wrote aimless essays at a table facing the sea. The rain dimpled the water all morning, washed away the afternoons, grumbled through the night. Everyone said it was the coldest, rainiest summer they could remember. I asked my parents to mail me my winter coat and deleted my Facebook account because pictures of friends in sundresses made me weep.

I was twenty-five, had forgotten how to make friends, had five months of nothing to do. In the afternoons, I read novels alone at a cinnamon-scented, subterranean coffeeshop where people around me talked of their purposeful lives—crabbing and parenting, hunting, art-making, and flying. I had no job, no children, no purpose but to wonder what mine was. Even on sunny days, surrounded by Sitka's searing beauty, I felt entitled to better: I couldn't hike because there was a bear every square mile. (Groups of three are generally exempt from attacks, but I didn't have enough friends to constitute a group.) When I went to swim at the beach, sea lions growled and shone in the ocean, making the water an expansive, threatening tease.

I was unwilling to let time reveal place, thinking that Sitka's first impression was so severe, it could never fully change. I told Luke he'd brought me to a place he'd misrepresented; he had raved about it rather than anticipating my potential isolation. Luke was doing some commercial fishing, which meant he was gone for days at a time (and even when he's guiding, he leaves the house every morning before five).

"The people and this place are cold," I said to him on the bench of his boat, where I could tell he was both deeply saddened and alarmed. If I didn't share this love of place with him, including its challenges, maybe I wouldn't be able to share a life with him, either.

"I thought you'd love it here," he said.

"I do," I said, which was true. "But I'm so lonely, I don't know what to do."

My instinct was to flee. Luke begged me to stay. His hair, already so blond, was reaching a bleached white in the sun, and his face had taken on a tan and taut and weather-beaten thickness. I was madly in love with him and desperate to leave. I knew that if I gave up this easily, I was giving up on all the things he had spent the last ten years building for himself—a business, his own boat, in a place that was less consumerist, more legit, more Luke-like than anywhere I could picture.

So I stayed. Not because of Alaska's here-then-gone beauty or Luke's quiet convincing but because of my own vanity: I didn't want to seem like a wuss to this man of steadfast integrity. Sometimes you have to fake strength to achieve it. I gained fifteen pounds that summer, eating fried halibut and tartar sauce and reading books indoors.

Every year I flew to Alaska, I was stunned by Sitka's grandeur and surprised I could still feel such a longing to be somewhere—anywhere—else. Every year I made maybe one new friend. One wife of a fisherman, also seasonal in Sitka, told me it had taken her thirteen years to make a single one.

I did make friends with Alaskans elsewhere, though. That first summer, as part of a graduate program in nonfiction writing, I left Sitka to read and write for two weeks in Anchorage, where the temperatures reached a balmy seventy degrees, and I met a friend who understood. Her name was Sara Loewen, and her husband fished, too. Only she had it worse: during fishing season, Sara and Pete and their infant son lived on an island with *no one else*. Every May, she took a small plane from Kodiak (where they live the rest of the year) to Uyak Bay with fifty-pound bags of flour, sugar, and rice, since at their setnet fish site, there are no stores. There Sara tended to a big garden and her dog and a handful of ducks, while brown bears combed the beach below the cabin the couple had built for themselves. The isolation crushed her, the beauty conflicted with her daily dream of leaving.

So Sara and I spent two weeks giggling like children in Anchorage, finding all the bookstores, running from moose on campus, drinking beers in crowded bars. When we left each other, we cried, knowing the loneliness that was waiting back in the land of fishing laundry and husbands who fall asleep during dinner. When I returned to Sitka, I cried every time I read her work because with solidarity came the permission to say *this is hard*.

We don't always say something's hard when it's happening. One of these times is when you're holding your brand-new child. Now, as I step off the airplane in Sitka with my daughters and my mom, I try to summon the calm that's expected of me, of all new moms. I know I'll see my hard-earned friends waiting for loved ones in the airport, that they'll want to see the baby, that they'll have no idea of the battle I'm already fighting between what people can see and what I feel to be true: that my child needs more than I or this place can provide. Looking out at the island's shimmering severity—blinding snow on sharp mountain peaks, the vastness of the water past where we can see—I know Alaska might wreck me again.

The day after we arrive, I have what Sara calls a "grace day" because

Luke has the day off. He's just done his commercial salmon fishing, cranking up twenty- and thirty-pound king salmon on his hand-troll equipment, so he's actually on land for a three-day stretch—his one "long" break of the season. We can have coffee together, I can shower without someone screaming in the bathroom—plus, praise God, there is sun!

It's a perfect day. I wear the one tank top I brought for the summer, we leave Anna with my mom, and we walk to the Fourth of July food booths downtown. Luke holds my hand, Zaley gets her face painted like a fish, and we eat Indian fry bread and play carnival games out of the 1950s. Later, in the afternoon, I stay home, marveling with my mom at Anna's multicolored eyes and her impossibly slender neck, while Luke fishes with Zaley in the high, waving grasses of the estuary. And later still, when everyone is asleep and the light is still bright, I sneak away and stroll the gravel trails in Totem Park, breathing in the wet scent of rust-colored cedars in a deadfall forest as dark as dusk.

The whole weekend feels dreamy, and because we still don't have the results for Anna's test, it's beginning to feel like maybe she doesn't have a disease.

But then it's Monday. I wait all day for Dr. Kono to call, and every time I think of him, my stomach feels like a pot being banged with a spoon. On Tuesday, I can't eat. So I call him instead. It's noon, sunny again, and Zaley and I are kicking a soccer ball out front.

Susie answers the nurse's line. "Megan. Hi." The *hi* plops out of her mouth, no lilt. "I don't have the authority to tell you the test results, sweetheart," she says. "But Dr. Kono is going to call you tonight from home."

I thank her, shaken, and hang up. *Call me from home? That must mean Anna has CMV. Or maybe she has something else.*

The phone rings again.

"Screw the rules, babe," Susie says. "I have to tell you. The test came back positive. Anna tested positive for congenital CMV."

The ball rolls past me, down the dirt driveway, and into the eddies of our berry-lined creek.

"Mom, you missed it!" Zaley is yelling. "Mom! Did you even see it? You just missed the ball!"

All the mountains on Baranof Island are at risk of sliding during heavy onslaughts of rain. Most of their slopes have been scarred by mud-brown chutes—permanent sutures that sound no alarm before they cut downhill.

I feel like what's left after a landslide. Mostly it's this word *progressive* that fells me. It means that nothing is stable, that I will be keeping vigil. Forever.

Dr. Kono does call that night and expresses that the first step is to obtain Anna's antiviral immediately. But all his other words lift straight out of the pages of my memory; phrases and details, in shock, take flight.

I am left with an image: a sphere, with spikes, blasting through Anna's bloodstream unendingly. The virus, every second I breathe, is penetrating one of Anna's pristine cells, using that cell's machinery to copy itself, then erupting outward to seek and infect the next. I cannot stand that this process is happening in real time, at a rate I can neither conceive of nor see. I don't really understand what a virus actually is. I know it isn't autonomous—or even really alive—because it needs a host to replicate and survive. But it isn't dead, either. It is a paradox. A haunting. I hate it more than I've hated anything in my life.

And to make matters worse, all I can do is what I always do in Alaska: wait. The sun is a blanched coin, taunting from the sky like it's late afternoon, while in reality, it's after five. Pharmacies anywhere east of Sitka are already closed.

Much later, after the haze of shock and sorrow have bled into night, I'm in bed. There's the velvet brown of our bedspread, the crackle of Luke snoring, the warmth of Anna's breath as her body fights and rests. In the last dregs of light, around midnight, I can still see the long shadows of Anna's already long eyelashes, and I run my index finger along them, watching them bend and return, like the pliable but unbreaking tines of a comb. In my body is an all-consuming love and an obliterating agony. Insomnia and a bone-deep need for sleep. A total aloneness and a total togetherness with this child who is disease and daughter all mixed together, and it seems like, if I think hard enough about it, maybe I can separate one from the other—cure her of her beginnings by understanding what I could have done differently.

Usually when people speak of "magical thinking," they're referencing death and the wish to bring a loved one back to life. As Joan Didion writes, after her husband has just died: "There was a level on which I believed that what had happened remained reversible." I feel like Didion, like this can't really be. But I can feel the pulse of something underneath the grief and that pulse is the drumbeat of guilt—can you grieve someone who's still alive, whom you love *unconditionally*—that is, without changing their *condition*? Does it make me a terrible person if I wish to bring back the child we'd imagined, the one who now will never be? I do love Anna as she is, but I want her to have an unfettered future, which seems to necessitate setting her free from this invasive component she contains.

Like Didion, I feel entitled to the life my mind had created, not the more complicated life we all end up having to live.

———

That first night, inside the battered new reality of congenital CMV, I know I should sleep. But instead I reach over to the nightstand for my computer and place it gently on the bed, opening it slowly since Anna wakes to light. I'm looking for the impossible: a glimpse of who Anna might one day be. I'm preoccupied with the possibility that everything I know about her could be taken from me—that her eyes could stop seeing, her mouth could cease nursing, her breath could desist. I want proof of the opposite: that she will progress and subvert the progressiveness of her disease. I also want to see what the speed of CMV's progressions can be.

In the time between Anna's test and Anna's diagnosis, a new website has come into existence: NATIONAL CMV FOUNDATION appears in royal blue on the screen. I click on it, and its banner ignites every follicle of my skin: *91% of American women have never heard of CMV.*

I feel like I'm in a movie, a movie barely anyone has seen. A simple thought rings out at high volume in my head, and it will change the rest of my life: This is not okay.

The tabs on the National CMV Foundation website read: PREG-

NANCY, PREVENTION, OUTCOMES, and STORIES. The PREGNANCY and PREVENTION tabs are too painful to touch. Like the CDC's page on CMV, all this information is invisible to the CMV-unaware world. Before I click anything, the homepage offers a ratio for how many children are born with CMV in America every year: *one in 200 babies*, it says. I do a double take: they must have meant one in 2,000 or something. I scroll around to find I am wrong.

My finger quivers over the OUTCOMES tab, and with eyes shut, I click it. I open one eye at a time to an ombré spectrum of symptoms: on the far right, in light aquamarine, are the words *No visible delays or impairments*. On the left, in a saturated teal, are the worst: *Miscarriage, Stillbirth, Infant or Child Loss*. In a new tab—because this is how I research CMV, with a need and greediness for all the information at once—I Google "stillbirth from CMV." The first link that appears is a 2011 study titled, "Have We Overlooked Congenital Cytomegalovirus as a Cause of Stillbirth?" in which the author firmly concludes yes: with 50 percent of stillbirths resulting from an infection during pregnancy, CMV greatly outnumbers any other pathogen in the placentas of stillborn infants.

Like everything I will read written by CMV specialists, this study is not just numbers and statements; this doctor is lobbying for major systemic change.

I go back to the National CMV Foundation because I still want to *see* CMV. The STORIES tab opens a Pandora's box of personal narratives accompanied by photographs. Here are children I will never forget. One of them, a girl named Bailey, is in Alaska, surrounded by her parents and her sister and what looks like a doctor in a hospital hallway. Bailey's hands are up near her chest, floppy at the wrists. While most children with CMV will live typical-length lives, four hundred will die every year from congenital CMV. Bailey died at the age of eighteen.

I keep scrolling, hungry to see more. Some children have a turned-in eye, while others have yellowing teeth. (CMV can cause ocular strabismus and destroy a child's dental enamel.) Some are spending their lives in wheelchairs, have seizures every hour, and have never slept through the night at the age of twenty-three. And then there are older kids who are unaffected-looking, graduating from college, and standing on their own two feet. I linger on these stories, but the narratives keep coming, and so does my grief. The asymptomatic kids' stories aren't comforting; they only make the spectrum of CMV seem longer and blurrier and more unjust.

I am moving down the page more quickly now, paying no respect to the individuality of each narrative. I'm desperate. I'm looking, I realize, for pictures of babies. Do some of the babies look like Anna and then end up not being able to walk? Do some of the babies who die look typical at birth?

Yes, they do. They look *normal*—a word I know I shouldn't use, but it's true. They look alert, excruciatingly oblivious, while incubating this invisible monster illness. Anna is asleep next to me in the bed, and I place a hand on her back to reassure myself she's still there, still respirating, still a baby who is mine and not these. I'd wanted the babies online to look more afflicted. I'd wanted to see that their limbs had come out gnarled or their eyes askew. I know it's perverse and unfair, but I've been looking for any sign that Anna could possibly be *not them*.

With a snap, I see that this is the problem. Couldn't any of these children be mine? And isn't this how I should have approached child-making in the first place—with the acceptance that anything at all could happen, with an awareness of our inevitable vulnerability? I slow way down. I go back up to Bailey and read what her mother wrote:

> She was social without communicating.
> She loved without words.
> She never seemed to want more than what was at her
> fingertips.
> When we put her arms around our necks, she used every
> tiny muscle in her body to hold on as tight as she could.
>
> I know she's already gone, but I don't want them to lose her.

———

There's a reason I'm seeking the stories of specific people—of even just one little girl: it's a concept called *entitativity*. Entitativity (one of the clunkiest words in the English language) means the inability to grasp, with feeling, a coherent picture of a situation you're trying to conceive. Unfortunately, we have a propensity to respond oppositely, with something known as "compassion fade"; historically, we respond to mass tragedies with little interest, even apathy, as soon as our perception of an event extends beyond impacting an individual into impacting many.

Renowned psychologist Paul Slovic looks at how this could be. While he focuses mostly on genocides, he proposes that the more we use numbers in any situation of human need—and the higher those numbers get—the more we are psychically numbed to any one disaster's effects. For example, when we hear the statistic "one million dead," our brain shuts itself down because it can't process this as an actual quantity or process the explosion of grief we'd feel if we could perceive of such a loss. Slovic calls this a "fundamental deficiency in our humanity" but suggests we can fix it by slowing down our thinking and focusing on specifics that pertain to an individual—their face, their eyes, their surroundings, their story. It's through this intimacy that we feel affect.

"One hypothesis might be that a single face creates empathy, which then motivates an action—a donation or some other kind of help," Slovic says. "But with a group, you may not get a clear picture, so you don't get the same response." In one of his studies, for example, the test subjects can donate to one child or to eight unrelated children who need lifesaving treatment. Participants end up giving far more to the single child than they do to the larger group.

Slovic and his colleagues suggest, though, that when several children are perceived to be in a coherent unit (by appearing in the same photograph or by being described as a family), the effect is comparable to viewing a single individual in need. Perceiving a suffering group as being intimately connected, then, may be a way of combating our inherent complacency in the face of crises.

"Ultimately," Slovic concludes, "thoughtful deliberation . . . may be necessary to alert us to an undesired disconnect between the high value we place on individual lives and our neglect of populations at risk."

✥

Luke wakes up, as though he knows what I'm doing. He clicks my computer closed and puts it on his nightstand, out of reach. He wraps his arm around me, careful not to bump the baby. I kiss his thick hand, then kiss Anna's spindly, purple-tipped fingers, each and every one. I think of that phrase *ten fingers and ten toes*—the line people always use to reference a wholly formed child, as though babies absent senses, digits, and abilities wouldn't garner the same kind of wonder. I love Anna explosively, maybe even more so because of her susceptibility. I nestle between their two hearts, and soon sleep settles over me on a night I thought it never would.

I dream without sound. I dream of a plane bringing medicine through fog.

———

Later that night Anna paws me awake to nurse, as she has since day one. She sleeps next to me all night and wakes me by touch rather than by her own sound. When I open my eyes, she is looking straight at me and continues to do so, while holding absolutely still, for minutes on end. And because she is so close and so stunning and so undisturbed, I stroke her chin again and again, and I know, in the almost-dark of the middle of the night, that I have never had a love—for anything or anyone—so complex, so vigilant, so full of mystery.

5

There's barely any blood after Anna arrives, as though postpartum issues take sides, and this time they're inside her body, not mine. I want the opposite. I want to go back to when CMV was my problem. I want to know if there were signs of the virus—at prenatal appointments, in my medical records, hiding inside the nuances of each cold I caught. I obsess over the question: *Could that have been it?* This is how new CMV mothers exist: jumping back and forth between pregnancy and baby, memories and reality, probing the silence and searching for clues.

It was the fall of 2014, during the glorious, postfishing month of September, when I first found out I was pregnant with Anna. I bounced down our stairs and into Luke's home office, holding the positive pregnancy test in the air like a baton. We did the calculations on our fingers, she would be due in June, and Luke said, "Oh, shit." Another baby due during fishing season. He'd had the same reaction with Zaley. I knew he just needed a little time to digest.

That night at bedtime, unable as ever to keep a secret, I held Zaley's face between my hands and told her she was going to be a big sister. When she planted an ecstatic kiss on my lips, I kissed her right back. I knew what lay ahead: fasting from spicy tuna rolls and turkey sandwiches and wine. But it is not common sense or empirical pregnancy wisdom to avoid the mouths of our kids.

A week later there was no CMV brochure in my OB's waiting room where other toddlers were always scrambling over the white leather couches with their moms' water bottles, no CMV conversation during my exam while Zaley sat on the rolling stool reserved for the doctor and ran my Chapstick around her lips. I would have remembered; I would have kept my Chapstick in my pocket instead of my purse for the next nine months.

For the rest of the fall, I washed my hands as much as usual, went for walks, ate as healthy as I could. But then in winter, there was that unshakable, mono-like something that I'd gotten along with Zaley. We'd spent days on the couch next to each other, watching *Berenstain Bears* and drinking from whatever cup was closest to our hands.

Unlike other viruses that transmit through the air or on a grocery cart, you can only contract CMV through direct contact with it—meaning when urine or mucus or saliva (which has a much higher viral load than other bodily fluids) goes straight into your mouth. This is why mothers are so at risk of catching CMV: toddlers don't control their drool very well, CMV can live on surfaces for up to six hours, and we eat our children's food. I'm sure I kissed Zaley's snot-smeared face, finished her half-eaten toast; I was too fatigued to go get my own, and like many pregnant women, I believed it was fine to get a pedestrian virus while pregnant—that I'd be supplying the baby in utero with healthy antibodies if I caught my kid's cold.

I brought Zaley to the pediatrician on call who listened to her lungs, said it was just a nasty virus—we should drink fluids and rest. No mention of CMV, despite the fact that I was clearly pregnant and my toddler was dripping. Zaley got better quickly, but I couldn't sleep at all in the night. I was in the minority in that CMV actually made me feel like I was ill.

Marica remembers seeing me at church and thinking I looked even worse than I usually do during pregnancy. "This isn't pregnancy sick," she says I told her. "It's something worse, something else. I don't know what it is."

At my twenty-week anatomy scan, the sonographer clicked around on the screen, and I asked her to slow down so I could see the beauty of the interlocking vertebrae and the hinge of each wrist. I also told her I'd been pretty sick. The tech said, curtly, "'Tis the season," then told me to look away. (Luke always insists on knowing if we're having a boy or a girl, and I always refuse.) I didn't want her to spill the news, so I shut my mouth, figured I was fine, played the obedient patient even though I really wanted to drown myself in Nyquil every night. There was nothing to see on the ultrasound at that point, even though CMV was likely already working its way toward Anna's ears and brain.

A few days after that, still feeling terrible, I called my OB. And that's when the nurse called back and said, "If you're that sick, then you shouldn't come in." She also said: "You should call your primary care doctor and ask for some meds."

Had I gone in, I now know, a midwife or an OB could have tested me for CMV.

———

The CMV test during pregnancy is a simple blood test, but the results can be complex. This is one reason OBs in the United States don't routinely test healthy pregnant women for CMV—a stance I will come to agree with in the years to come.

It does, however, make sense to request a test for CMV if a pregnant woman is experiencing a long-lasting illness (as I did) or if there's evidence of fetal abnormalities on ultrasound. The scenario plays out in my head: if the doctors had tested me shortly after I was sick, they might have found evidence of short-term antibodies to CMV in my system—which may have indicated a recent infection.

Alternately, they might have found no short-term antibodies but long-term antibodies with what's called "low avidity," meaning my antibodies had just recently switched from short-term to long-term and the infection was recent enough to be dangerous to my fetus.

Or they may have found both short-term *and* long-term antibodies to CMV in my system. Which is where it gets a little tricky.

Often doctors will look at a CMV test and assume that because a woman has long-term antibodies to CMV, she carries immunity to it and she's "safe." However, this is not entirely the case. There are thousands of strains of CMV, so a woman can always be *reinfected* with a previously uncontracted strain. Meaning no one is immune to CMV, and all pregnant women are at risk—a lesson not often messaged to women even when they receive a test.

It is true that these reinfections—and also *reactivations* of a latent form of CMV in a woman's body—cross the placenta only about 1 percent of the time, as opposed to 30 to 40 percent of the time if a woman is experiencing a more serious first-time or *primary* case of

CMV. But these nonprimary infections from reinfection or reactivation do still lead to substantial caseloads of congenital CMV: in poorer, more populated countries where the vast majority of women have already had CMV long before pregnancy, they're giving birth to just as many babies with congenital CMV.

In an ideal world, if I'd been tested and was suspected of having either a primary or a nonprimary CMV infection, I might have had a conversation with my doctor. I might have had more frequent ultrasounds. I might have understood the importance of obtaining immediate treatment if she were to be symptomatic and test positive at birth. I may even have been registered in a clinical trial and been treated with antivirals during pregnancy, which can diminish the power of a virus and stop it from populating the placenta by reducing its viral load.

But there's also the alternative: What if the virus I had right then wasn't CMV? What if I'd had *no* antibodies to CMV and I'd been educated about where it lurked? What if I'd still had a chance to prevent contracting the disease because I knew what it was?

Like many women my age, I didn't have a primary care physician—I saw my OB for everything I needed. So I called my dad's PCP. No matter that he specialized in geriatrics; I'd seen him before, and he could see me that day. I begged for codeine, knowing it was a category C pregnancy drug (not recommended unless the benefit outweighs the risk) and knowing I needed something effective so I could work and sleep and still be nice to Zaley. My mom and Luke were taking turns watching her during the fishing off-season while I ran a nonprofit writing program in the Denver public school system for kids from fifth through twelfth grade. The doctor said he'd write me the script, and the choice was up to me.

I filled the codeine prescription, took it for a few nights, and slowly returned to what seemed normal health and sleep. My close friend Mia was also pregnant with her second baby. Her first daughter was Zaley's age, Zaley's best friend, and she was in daycare—where nearly 80 percent of young children will contract a CMV infection within two years. After Mia picked her daughter up from daycare, we'd get together and share pregnancy gripes, trade tantrum stories, and dip pretzels into the same hummus container as the girls.

I'll never know if Zaley had CMV or if her friend did. Nor do I want to. "I think diseases have no eyes," Sandra Cisneros wrote in *The House on Mango Street*, a book I always used while teaching high school students how to write about tough things. "They pick with a dizzy finger anyone, just anyone." I do believe diseases land with a whirling randomness, which is one reason I've never felt contracting CMV was any child's fault or only the fault of my own.

The other reason is that to know how to prevent a disease, the medical field has to disclose that it exists.

6

In the house where we live in Sitka, seven tall windows face the sea. Below these windows is a soft brown couch, and this is where I sit, nursing Anna and directing Zaley for hours of the day. In between games and requests and negotiations, I always look over my shoulder at the roil of the water. I'm trying to catch that moment before the wave pattern changes, before the water becomes whiter or blacker or bluer than it was a minute earlier. But I can't—the surface changes before I realize it's changing, every time.

I turn to Anna as often as I turn to the waves, searching her eyes, their color-streaked depth, for any precursor of change. I'm looking for signs of chorioretinitis—floaters, redness, leaking—which can be caused by CMV and could make my daughter go blind.

The thought of blindness is like an erasure in my brain. When I have my eyes up close to Anna's, scrutinizing, Zaley will tug at my neck and say, "Mom! Give her some space!" I never do see spots or floaters. All I can see is Anna's sharpness and clarity and the reflection of myself and Zaley across the gloss of her eyes. Anna's eyes are the source of my darkest worries, and yet, a wellspring of deep, silent calm.

"Life is this simple," writes Thomas Merton, the Trappist monk and prolific writer who sought temporary refuge from the noise of the world in Alaska. "We are living in a world that is absolutely transparent and the divine is shining through it all the time. This is not just a nice story or a fable, it is true."

***

The morning after Anna's diagnosis, I dial the hospital on Japonski

Island, which is a five-minute drive from our house, over the ten-story bridge and onto the chunk of forested land that houses the airport, Coast Guard base, and steam-producing, Communist-looking hospital. A nurse answers the line: "This is Jolene."

"My daughter," I say, and before the third word is out, my voice has gone high and trembly. "She's two weeks old and just got diagnosed with congenital CMV." There's a second, maybe two, of nothing. This silence has a meaning under it, as it always does: Jolene has never heard of my daughter's disease. "Our pediatrician in Colorado said we need to get her on a drug as soon as possible to preserve her hearing and her brain."

"Hold on just a minute," she says. Jolene has a slow, understanding voice, a drawl not of Southernness but of kindness, and I can feel she's concerned and listening. I will look for this audible compassion in every provider we see.

A click, and she's back: "Can you come first thing in the morning?"

———

I wake to the rasp of rain on the window screen, the quiet clucks of the chickens next door. I get out of bed gently enough to not wake the baby, and I walk to the kitchen table, where Zaley is already having tea with my mom. Outside is a layer cake of fog. I can hear the rainwater on the deck, like a hundred pricking needles, and I want to run away.

Instead, I fill my coffee cup and bring it back to the bedroom to get dressed. I'm still tiptoeing around, sneaking into jeans and a sweater as though Anna might be able to hear me. She's awake now on the bed, bringing her fists under her chin, squinting, and arching her back. She does so many typical baby things. I say a prayer that has no words—it's just an all-out, eyes-shut, silent, internal shrieking.

Zaley sneaks into the room and pulls herself onto the bed. She leans over Anna, whispers into her ear: "Can you hear me, baby? I'm going to do puzzles with Nana and wait for you right here."

I zip my burnt-orange raincoat over the slightest bump where Anna used to live, pick her up, and walk hand in hand with Zaley to the door. My mom, my safety net, takes Zaley's hand as soon as I let it go. She stands with her in a dry circle on the porch while I shuffle

Anna out to the car. Then Zaley waves madly till I drive out of sight.

———

There are problems with our car. It's a giant, rusted-out, white Chevy Suburban, and anytime it rains, the brakes audibly jam and grind, so descending our steep dirt driveway toward the street is a daily exercise in ceding control. "Please work, please work," I implore aloud on the way down our hill. Usually, the brakes catch well enough for me to mostly stop at the stop sign, and if not, I can fake a rolling stop/overzealous left turn and coast the rest of the way to the main road into town.

Today I'm in good shape. But as soon as we veer right onto Sawmill Creek, Anna remembers she hates the car. I can hear her screaming, but I cannot see her. I start singing to her, but the sound of my voice brings me closer to the bad thing: *What if she doesn't know I'm here because she can't hear me at all?* Because the car is as long as a boat, I can't reach back and touch her. Even though the ride is a tenth of what it would be at home, each minute reminds me how hard it is to see and treat her needs.

We cross the bridge and the wave-laced channel below, where painted boats are bringing fish to the seafood co-op and a floatplane is pushing back into the center of the water. I pass the dormitories of Mount Edgecumbe High School, where teenagers from villages all over Alaska come to live and learn. Then I turn right at the hospital sign and angle into a parking spot with a loud metallic lurch. When I open the car door, the rain feels even harsher here on this smaller island, where the water is closer on every side. So I unzip my coat, put Anna upright against my chest, then zip her inside the waterproof fabric before racing us up the stairs.

Inside, it smells like warm cafeteria food, and Anna is quiet. I leave her inside my coat and push the elevator button, which gives off a more cheerful ding than it seems like it should. On the second floor, at the receptionist's window, I give a nurse our name. She smiles at the top of Anna's head, says, "So much hair!" and walks us to a pediatric exam room to wait.

I'm relieved. Instead of idealized photographs on the walls, there are painted pink jellyfish, seaweed, and spouting blue whales. I'm also grateful for the lack of music. And when the pediatrician walks in, my chest unlatches and expands: he's older, not a young parent who's going to tell me about his own unafflicted kids. Dr. Vastola has a gray beard, glasses, and grown children, and I recognize him from lunchtime lap swimming at the Blatchley Pool in summers past.

"So this is Anna," he says, smiling. "Congratulations!"

This initial, genuine kindness about brings me to the floor. Then he takes her from my hands like the veteran baby-holder he is, with one hand under her bottom and one under her neck and head. He brings her near his face. "To be honest," he says, "she looks so asymptomatic, I don't think I would have tested her for CMV."

While Dr. Vastola continues to examine Anna with the slowest motions, he says—as Dr. Kono did—that he's never actually seen a child with CMV. Statistically, I figure they both probably have and just don't know it. I picture the kids in both places who have cerebral palsy or late-onset hearing loss, glasses or unexplained cognitive delays. Actually, I am constantly picturing the other kids with CMV. I feel that if I can conceive of their existence—and their numbers—it will help validate Anna's diagnosis, which I still seem to be experiencing in a dark and silent vacuum.

Exactly one year later, a sizable chunk of America will see CMV, though most won't realize it: Marlana VanHoose, a petite young woman the size and likeness of a ten-year-old, will stand in front of the Republican National Convention with her dark brown bob and opaque, red-lensed sunglasses and stun the audience with her rendition of the national anthem. In truth, Marlana is twenty years old when she performs; she is tiny, blind, and has cerebral palsy from congenital CMV. The audience won't ever hear the letters CMV, though—they'll identify the most noticeable thing, which is that the singer can't see. They won't have a name for the invisible virus that caused her growth restriction, her loss of sight, her curled left hand.

"I'm going to have to do some research tonight," Dr. Vastola continues, laying Anna down and pressing on her abdomen to see if she has abnormalities in her lungs or spleen. "The most important thing is that we get this antiviral into her system quickly. The success rate of Valtrex is based on starting it within the next week. Problem is, the drug isn't even close to available here."

When he gets to Anna's chest, he notices what I have, too: her nipples and the flesh surrounding them are raised by nearly an inch, as if tiny breakfast patties were floating under her skin. "This is the most impressive breast tissue I think I've ever seen," Dr. Vastola says. "It's probably just hormonal—induced by the hormones in your milk. But I think maybe she should see an endocrinologist, too. CMV can cause precocious puberty from damage to her pituitary gland."

This is news. What he means is that CMV can cause little girls to have their periods as toddlers or very young girls. The thought of this is a blunt hammer to my heart. It seems like CMV can cause, basically, everything.

Next, his fingers stop on her sternum. "Boy," he smiles, "she sure is a cutie."

She is. And though it's the smallest comment, I start to cry. Because of all the things he has noticed about Anna, he also sees something he might see in any other child. While I wipe my eyes, he says she has good flexibility in her limbs, that they're low-toned but not overly stiff. "We will need an ultrasound of her brain, which I think we can do here," he adds. "And we're going to have to gold-streak the medication from Juneau. If your insurance approves it."

"Gold-streak?" I ask.

"It means we have to find a small plane to fly it here as soon as it arrives in Juneau. It's a liquid and must be kept at a certain degree. If it sits there overnight, it could be ineffective by the time it reaches her."

I think of the hospital in Denver—how we could have walked two minutes down the hallway to get her medicine, had I been tested during pregnancy because of her smallness, or had she been tested because of her failed hearing tests, right after birth.

And then it's like *If You Give a Mouse a Cookie*: when I think of Denver, I think of flying home. When I think of flying, I think about the shadow a plane makes on the surface of the ocean. When I think about the ocean, I think about Luke. And then I'm sunk. I miss the heat of his body next to mine at these appointments. (And in Alaska, he's always too hot because he wears his thick fleece Grundéns that keep his body at one hundred-plus degrees.) I miss the cushion that he is in every situation of stress. Sometimes, he's so stable it can feel minimizing of my concerns, but now I wouldn't even mind that. If he were here, he'd be listening and squeezing my hand and saying, "Well . . . shit," and just his voice would rebuild some of the ruin.

Dr. Vastola is still talking, listing all the therapies and specialists Anna will need during early childhood, and the quantity is dizzying: to begin with, she'll need an infectious disease team, a neurologist, an audiologist, an ophthalmologist, an endocrinologist, a speech pathologist, an occupational therapist, a physical therapist, and the good old pediatrician. *Holy crap,* I'm thinking. *This all basically came from a cold.* I'm also not writing anything down.

The land of writing, of pens and notebooks and the privilege of putting the world's details on a page, feels like an alternate universe—a place from which this illness has permanently exiled me. With all of Anna's needs, how will I possibly ever write again?

"Valgancyclovir," Dr. Vastola explains, unaware of the existential crisis I'm having in my mind, "is an oral drug we'll use for the next six months. Because it can cause the bones to stop producing marrow, we'll need baseline bloodwork, then weekly blood draws to monitor her white blood cells."

"Baseline bloodwork, meaning we need her blood right now?"

"Yes," he answers. "The lab is just down the hall." He is snapping Anna's onesie around her one-inch thighs. "Make sure you ask for Jerry. They're going to have a hard time with her veins."

I take Anna from Dr. Vastola and thank him with a voice so overwhelmed, it barely makes any noise. Then I carry Anna down the clean, windowed hall as if we're not ourselves but characters cast in a bizarre novel without dialogue or sound. We pass a friend of mine, a poet from grad school who is also there with her daughter, and she leans in to admire Anna. I linger for a moment, but when she asks if everything's okay, I shake my head, cannot speak. I know she understands that words are not always as powerful as our feelings. I feel like a boat full of water, as if one more particle might trigger my slow descent.

I look out the rain-dashed windows for a minute before entering the lab. The rain is the sideways kind from which you cannot shield yourself or your child—not with your hands, not with an umbrella, not with the rain gear I haven't even unpacked. I feel that I cannot protect Anna from anything.

7

Jerry is on vacation. Two nurses have me sit in a motorized chair with turquoise pads. Thankfully, I'm allowed to nurse while they try to draw Anna's blood. But the first jab to her heel sends her into such a rage, feeding is impossible. The second poke enters her violet-lined wrist, and I can tell it has missed. The purple is pooling under her skin, and the room tightens with frustration. Five more people pierce her in five other places, unsuccessfully, until I have memorized the contours of Anna's gums, the pattern of vibrations her tongue makes when she screams.

Finally, an hour later, an IV-renowned nurse practitioner from the ER comes up and successfully pulls blood from Anna's *scalp,* which I didn't even know was possible. I feel so responsible. How could I hold her and allow this torture? Now I'm crying harder than Anna, and I don't even care. Saint Isaac the Syrian once described tears as the border between the bodily and the spiritual state, and this does feel like an intersection of realms, as if the protective barrier between how I feel and how I look were finally coming down.

A graduate professor of mine, Eva Saulitis, had written about something similar before she died too young for anyone around her to accept it with the grace she did. Eva was a marine biologist who wrote about "thin places"—where the material world exists in close proximity to the spiritual world. She focused on physical geography, Prince William Sound and its orca whales specifically, but sitting here sobbing with Anna—who's now quiet in my arms—I wonder if the sick reside closer to where it's thin, where the line between the earthly and the otherworldly falls away. I remember the way Anna looked, her very first day, how her eyes seemed to seek somewhere that was not here.

———

The nurses are applying too-big Dora the Explorer Band-Aids all over their mistakes, and I am begging them to stop because these, too, will hurt Anna when I peel them off at home. A woman appears in dark pink scrubs. She's the lab director, and she's embarrassed. She asks for my email address: for all the trouble they've had with Anna's IV, she's gifting us with a hundred-dollar certificate to a toy store online. Only in a small town do we receive this kind of genuine apology or acknowledgment.

And apologies in the field of medicine, I will soon learn, are both rare and of more importance than many health professionals realize.

When I get home, I can't think of anything, ironically, that Anna could need. So I use the certificate to buy Zaley a Melissa & Doug castle complete with yarn-tailed horses, fabric queens, and a wooden drawbridge that lifts and lowers on hinges of thread. I've been saying no to everything Zaley asks me to do with her: no to going to the Science Center to pet the anemones; no to building Zaley a dollhouse made from the discarded Amazon boxes like we built last summer. "Now you'll have a castle," I tell her, showing it to her online. We didn't make it together, but it's pink instead of brown, and all its upper edges have those toothy, crenellated edges I never could have made myself. I realize it might feel like a summer of saying no, but maybe it isn't. Maybe it's a season of learning a different yes.

That night I write. I'm too tired to do it, but I write anyway. I've had a blog for years where I've shared photos of Alaska with friends and family down south. Maybe I can direct people here when they have questions and I don't have the energy to answer. Maybe I can save another CMV mother from the loneliness I feel.

———

As though reading my mind, the next morning, my mom asks: "How are you going to tell people what she has?"

I tell her I've written about it. But when I go to email friends and family members the basics, it hits me that the basics are too complex, that I really have no answers, just this big, bad CMV bomb to drop on everyone we know. And a number of my friends—and two of my sisters-in-law—on the email chain are pregnant.

I realize that I shouldn't be disclosing CMV to them for the first time; their doctors should be. And while I can write all night on my blog about how I feel, I don't yet understand CMV enough to address all the practical questions people will have: Contagiousness? Treatment? Testing during pregnancy? The dreaded question: Will Anna be okay? I can't bear articulating that I have no answer to that.

I wish I could read a book about what I'm going through, recommend it to friends. Books have been the most abundant and calming aspect of my life. They've also been my roadmap toward what is worth knowing. As one of my favorite writers, Susan Orlean, wrote: "Books are a sort of cultural DNA, the code for who, as a society, we are, and what we know."

But I can find only one book about CMV, called *Stealth Virus,* and it was written by a virologist, not by a mother. And because it was self-published in the UK, it will take at least a week to arrive. CMV clearly isn't a part of who we are and what we know, even though up to 80 percent of us already contain it in our bodies, and it's been in existence since animals with backbones started to evolve.

My mom can see that I'm struggling to write my email's first line. So while she suits up Zaley for their twenty-minute stroll to the mailbox, I open a few of the medical articles about CMV I haven't yet read. This time, phrases leap out: *global public health crisis* and *urgent action is required* and *a pregnancy epidemic, largely ignored.*

Crisis? Urgent? Epidemic? Ignored? Part of me wants to doubt the imperative of these words—because I read a lot and have doctors as family members, I believe we would have known. But I also suspect infectious disease doctors would not have written these phrases if they weren't true. I can feel the pounding of my heartbeat when I read, in one study, a chilling corroboration of Dr. Vastola's confession that he wouldn't have tested Anna for the disease: in the United States, according to health insurance claims data, even when CMV symptoms are present at birth, fewer than 10 percent of these newborns are tested for the condition. Which means that even when CMV is visible, doctors are missing it, and the vast majority of children affected by CMV are missing the window for treatment.

A thought flashes by that someone or some entity might be keeping this information from people—from pregnant women, specifically—but I don't have time to chase it. I can hear Zaley chirping up the hill, and I need to finish this email and hit send.

Minutes after I do, the emails come flooding back. People are upset, consoling, crying, concerned. But the one I will carry closest to my heart is from Luke's aunt—Anita's sister, Lynne. Her son, Bob, is undergoing his thirtieth surgery to fix a congenital condition that resulted in him being born without a complete esophagus. Lynne tells me not to believe any predictions placed upon Anna's life.

She writes that after Bob was born, his doctors said he would never ride a bike. So her husband went and found the biggest, shiniest bike for him to ride—which Bob eventually did. They said Bob would never be taller than five feet. Now he's six foot two. They said he'd be "severely mentally retarded." Now he has two college degrees and supports himself entirely.

But the next thing she writes sticks with me. She says, with authority: "Guard your imagination."

I'd imagined two daughters playing together in the yard. I'd imagined a tea party, a table, two chairs. I know that Anna could make it through this with only hearing loss, but even so, my mind keeps going to the place that is still and dark. When I read Lynne's email, I picture a gate, the sound of it locking down. Inside the gate is that scene: cups, spoons, and saucers. Two girls, one smaller than the other. I'm not close enough to see any hearing aids, to hear the sound of their chatter. When I'm being good, I don't rattle the gate. I stand diligent, outside its doors. There are two girls, and this is enough.

PART II

CONTEMPLATION

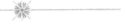

"The greatest kindness one can render to any man consists in leading him from error to truth."

SAINT THOMAS AQUINAS

I

I'm in the children's section of the library, facing the same sea and mountains we can see from the house. The fog today is ropelike, two threads woven around a nameless, uninhabited island in the sound. The sea is ice-colored, broken at its surface by the thrashing black heads of sea lions who prowl for carcasses tossed off the backs of boats. Between nursing Anna and asking Zaley not to pull twenty books off each shelf, I'm scanning each boat for Luke's—for the thick maroon stripe across the top, the reddish shine of the name *Drifter* across the bow.

Because the library faces the runway, I'm also watching the planes, imagining all the places you can go if you leave this forested rock. I would go to Colorado for its mainstream hospitals, Target, the sun. But I can't quite conceive of leaving. To leave would feel like leaving the country. (There's a reason Alaskans say, "How was America?" when you travel to the Lower 48.)

Also, I associate leaving midseason with medical emergency. A friend of mine here has to fly to Seattle for a lumpectomy in her neck. Another is airlifted to Anchorage for a stomach infection and stones in his bladder. And a third is rushed to Seattle at the end of her pregnancy because her newborn is going to need open heart surgery. There's something so disconcerting to me about their departures, about my friends' recoveries in vacuous hotel rooms instead of their own cozy homes. I don't want to go to hotels and hospitals I've never seen, where CMV's reality will be delivered, test by test, chart by chart. Where I will, inevitably, be alone.

With Anna's bills already piling up and my return to work indefinitely delayed, there's no way Luke can take a single day off. I want to stay in Sitka and deal with things here. This might be called denial. But it's also the closest thing to loyalty I've ever felt for Alaska.

———

My friend walks into the library with her son, who's two. I haven't seen her yet this summer, and she wants to see the baby. Around the perimeter of her face is a paleness I can't place. Then it hits me. I know what she's going to say before she does: "I'm pregnant!"

I congratulate her. And then she asks to hold Anna.

I hesitate. I'm afraid to tell her what Anna has. No doctor has warned me of this situation—being in close proximity to a pregnant woman—even though now I'm kicking myself. I'm thirty-two years old; Anna is going to be around pregnant women for all her early years. I don't know how to handle this hazard. I do know that it won't help, as time goes on, to test Anna's saliva for CMV to see if she's still contagious—babies and toddlers who have CMV, whether congenitally or not, can be shedding the virus one day and not shedding it the next.

My friend is waiting. Anna is sleeping. I tell her yes.

And there they are. A healthy pregnant woman holding my perfectly innocent, contagious baby. She's so newly pregnant, she's not even showing. A first-trimester infection could devastate her pregnancy.

I know I should tell her about CMV, that I'm as silent as my doctors were when I was pregnant. I think of that line of Molière's: "It is not only what we do, but also what we don't do, for which we are accountable." I feel a complicity in this grave omission. I feel accountable to this silence now that I know it exists.

But I'm also weighing my responsibility against my exhaustion. If I add this can of worms to my day, if I end up getting into a heated discussion with my friend, I know I'll be compromising the energy I need just to get to bedtime. (I don't know yet that later, my friend will handle the CMV conversation with compassion and intelligent questions, like a champ.) But in the moment, in the library, I realize I'm not just feeling complicit; I'm feeling pissed.

Because alongside everything else I'm juggling, I should not have to educate every pregnant woman I meet about the most common intrauterine infection. What a giant, medical embarrassment to leave this topic to those of us who are already dealing with the daily burden of the disease. This subject should be discussed by our trained and trusted OBs, in a setting intended for medical consultations and questions, not on the floor of the already frenetic, sweat-inducing space of the children's library, which Zaley and my friend's son have now mistaken for a place to do loud gymnastics.

Anna is, mercifully, asleep. Her arms are swaddled, and she's tucked inside a restrictive, fleece sack. I know she probably won't sneeze. And she definitely won't pee through the three layers she's wearing, or sit up and plant a wet kiss on my friend's mouth. While Anna is a risk, the more likely one is my friend's son, who isn't a baby with contained fluids, who has hands that touch his mouth and books and toys and can spread germs around the room.

For now, in the library, I am beginning to feel something new and unsettling—a stigma unfairly associated with infectious disease: that because my daughter's condition is contagious, rather than genetic, we are somehow unclean.

As soon as Anna peeps, I take her back, and my relief is a wave, cold and hungry.

———

After my friend leaves the library, I stand with Anna by the window. We're so close to the glass, it feels cool. I look at the spine of the mountain across from ours. The tree-blackened landmass looks like a person laboring to pull something out of the water—the hunch of a back stooped in a position of forever effort. This is how I feel, head down, hoisting something up, its shape and heft still a mystery. And like that island—the one with old logging scars but no homes, forests but no smoke—the island of CMV is a place where I'm still living entirely alone.

I sit down on the purple bench under the window and take out my phone. I type the question that's been gnawing at me and that now, after seeing a pregnant friend, feels critical to know: *Do obstetricians ever discuss CMV with women?*

Something appears that I've not yet seen: it's a national bulletin published by ACOG—the American Congress of Obstetricians and

Gynecologists—this year, in 2015. I scroll through it and reach a section titled "How should women be counseled about prevention of cytomegalovirus?" That section begins with this sentence: "Some groups of women are at higher risk of CMV infection." Childcare workers, it explains. And mothers like me, who have a young child at home. Nonetheless, the next statement begins in a tone whose end I can already predict. "Some have suggested that pregnant women should be instructed on the importance of personal hygiene and safe-handling techniques"—such as rigorous handwashing after diaper changes and using your own silverware at meals. But then it reads: "Such guidelines may be difficult to implement because they often are considered impractical or burdensome."

Impractical or *burdensome?* My face is aflame. Basically, the bulletin is insinuating that OBs in America should not discuss CMV with pregnant patients, should not attempt the chance to prevent severe childhood disability and early childhood death, because washing our hands more vigorously would cause us too much distress. The final line in the paragraph reads: "At present, such patient instruction remains unproven as a method to reduce the risk of congenital CMV infection."

I read it twice, then three, then four times, in a stupor of disbelief. Avoiding saliva where a virus lives hasn't been *proven* as a way to reduce our risk?

I look to the bottom of the document next, to see what study has been conducted to verify the generalization they're making about women and what we find burdensome. But there are no footnotes, no data indicating that ACOG has collected any insights from actual women who believe simple protective measures would be an unbearable nuisance while safeguarding the most critical stages of the development of life.

———

In medicine, doctors sometimes invoke a controversial principle called "the therapeutic privilege," which basically permits physicians, in rare cases, to alter—or fully withhold—information when the disclosure of the information would cause a patient incapacitating mental distress. Also known as "benevolent deception," this practice uses a doctor's good intentions, or benevolence, to justify medical silence—to condone a well-meaning lie.

However, many doctors and their guiding agencies, including the American Medical Association, ban the use of therapeutic privilege. "Withholding medical information from patients without their knowledge or consent is ethically unacceptable," decided the American Medical Association's Council on Ethical and Judicial Affairs in 2010. *The Handbook of Clinical Neurology* echoes this position, stating that "the [doctor's] desire to avoid emotional suffering for the patient is not alone sufficient justification for withholding critical medical information."

Individual doctors who specialize in bioethics are likewise opposed to the practice of benevolent deception. According to Dr. Alan Meisel, a leading international authority on informed consent, information should be kept from patients "when, but only when, its disclosure would so upset a patient that he or she could not rationally engage in a conversation about therapeutic options and consequences."

Who knows what I would have done if I'd been counseled about CMV during my pregnancies? I might have been worried or incredulous. I might even have been superstitious, believing that because I'd heard of CMV, now it wouldn't happen to me (which might have proven true; knowing about CMV very likely does reduce your chances of contracting it). What I can say, with utter certainty, is that I still would have been able to "rationally engage in conversation."

But knowing what I know about ACOG's silence, I'm not so sure about keeping cool right now. I want to scream. Or smash the fish tank in my OB's office with a bat.

In the absence of the aquarium, my anger drives me to a more reasonable outlet: research. I pull out my time-buying card and tell Zaley she can pick out a movie from the library to bring home—which I know will take her ten minutes, maybe more. And then I look up whether other women feel the same about discussing CMV with their OBs.

I find a recent study, published in 2014, in which eight hundred women participated. All of them had young children and were either pregnant or hoping to conceive. All the women learned about CMV briefly through a fact sheet or a short video. The conclusion:

after learning about CMV, 90 percent of the participants wanted more information about the disease. Additionally, up to 95 percent "agreed" or "strongly agreed" that they would attempt the advised protective measures (avoiding contact with saliva while kissing their child; avoiding shared eating utensils; washing hands after changing a wet diaper or wiping a child's nose) to reduce their risk of contracting CMV. I feel both outraged and affirmed.

I click the back arrow and see that there's a slightly larger Italian study on the same subject. In it, about half of the women were told about CMV and how to avoid it at the beginning of their pregnancy. The other half of women were chosen at delivery, women who had never been counseled about CMV. In the end, women who hadn't been told were seven times more likely to contract CMV during pregnancy than those who'd been counseled about the disease. The lead author, Dr. Maria Revello, concludes that hygiene counseling "may represent a responsible and acceptable primary prevention strategy to reduce congenital CMV."

This is a horrific revelation: that five minutes of counseling might have saved us, saved Anna, from everything we are experiencing and are about to experience.

But as I'm reading the numbers, I realize I'm not even that interested in the causal relationship between behaviors and prevention, though this correlation does seem to exist; the truth I'm after is proof that women can handle the facts—no matter how inconvenient, no matter how complex.

The mothers in Dr. Revello's study didn't run screaming from information about CMV. Just as in the other study, after being counseled about CMV, 80 percent of women did their best to avoid CMV either "often" or "always." And 93 percent reported that CMV recommendations were worth publicizing to pregnant women. They didn't lose any bonding with their toddlers, they didn't resist change. They, too, wanted the truth.

Of course they did, I think, clicking the lock button on my phone and watching it go dark. For what else more fully guides us than seeking answers that are accurate and sincere? I look at the stack next to me, and Zaley has, as usual, picked out all nonfiction books from the shelves. I can't pin her choices fully on her own preferences, of course, since she knows nonfiction is what I read and write. But our affinity for honesty is undeniable. From theology to science, philosophy to medicine, childhood to adulthood, veracity is always the pinnacle we seek—and pregnancy, when our body is literally more capacious than at any other time in the span of human life, does not weaken our capacity to embody the truth.

———

Sitting in the library, I see that my initial question—*Do women want the truth?*—has a simple answer.

Maybe what I'm actually asking is: *Who gets to decide what we can handle?*

I certainly don't tell Zaley; she decides for herself. A cautious child by nature—though also paradoxically wild—she doesn't like planes taking off, the deep end of the pool, or performing in front of crowds. And yet given her own autonomy, she continues to undergo all of the above. It isn't easy for me to watch her test the limits of her comfort. But it's the right way to love.

2

Alaska is a place where surviving depends on being informed about risk. From the minute I arrived in Sitka, I knew I needed to learn how not to die.

My only friend, Natalie, became my informal wilderness guide. She'd been a teacher at Raven's Way, a rehab program for Alaskan youth battling substance abuse who, after detoxing in town, were taken to an unoccupied, bear-filled island where they had to survive, for days, completely alone. The program had high rates of success because confronting their total vulnerability didn't terrify them; it gave them self-reliance and strength.

On weekend mornings when both of our husbands were fishing, Natalie and I would hike the Cross Trail with a can of bear spray in one of our backpacks and a cattle bell attached to the collar of her fast black dog. She was more at peace between tall hedges than I ever was, as I quietly imagined what dark shadows could become. Natalie was content not because she didn't think about bears. It was the opposite: she carefully considered the ecosystem and its threats at all moments in time.

I, on the other hand, was scared because of what I didn't know. I wanted the knowledge Natalie had, and I asked her for it. She taught me which berries you can eat in "Southeast"—as Alaskans call the Alaskan Panhandle—and which plants to avoid, how to act big and loud if we ever saw a bear. I kept asking questions, we kept hiking, and I gradually grew less scared. I would end up doing some contract writing for the Sitka Conservation Society that summer, and after talking to the bear biologist in town, I learned an interesting thing I'd never considered: even though most people in Sitka don't want to have an encounter with a bear in the wild, the bears' presence here increases most people's quality of life.

What he was saying is that knowing of a threat wasn't too much for people to handle. Living with risk replaced complacency with awareness and diversity. The risks raised the stakes. The risks made life more worth living.

———

I decide, after leaving the library, that I need to call my OB. When the nurse answers the phone, Zaley is animatedly explaining ice cream pasteurization in the background thanks to one of her library books, and I don't have the heart to quiet her. Actually, I don't want to; I figure it was the doctor's unawareness of her existence during my pregnancy that likely landed me here in the first place. When a nurse puts the doctor on the phone, I tell him that Anna has CMV.

"I'm so sorry," he says. And in the few seconds of silence that follow, I can tell he's offering consolation for the way Anna is, not acknowledging that he could have done anything differently. Then he tacks on, "Especially because CMV is just so rare."

I bristle, then ask the question I'm here for: "Do you ever counsel any of your patients about CMV?"

"ACOG doesn't recommend it," he says quickly. "Plus, women won't want to worry about one more thing."

No inquiry of my opinion, even though, as a woman living the consequences of this assumption, I would have been the perfect person to ask.

———

One of my favorite doctors is a doctor I've never met. His name is Atul Gawande—a best-selling author and surgeon who writes unflinchingly about problems in the culture of medicine today, specifically that doctors are trained more in competence than in understanding their patients' long-term desires and emotional needs. Dr. Gawande has also functioned as a humble journalist, learning from chefs how they run the most efficient kitchens, how basketball coaches produce the most winning teams—and then applying these methods, often involving humility and teamwork, to the training of doctors.

In an address at Harvard University, where he's a professor, he told a group of students:

> What I found over time, trying to follow and emulate people that were focused on achieving something more than competence, is that they weren't smarter than anybody else, they weren't geniuses. Instead, they seemed to be people that could come to grips with their inherent fallibility—fallibility in the systems that they work in, and with what it took to overcome that fallibility.

> Unfortunately, he says, this trait is not alive and well in medical culture today. Doctors disclose their mistakes less than half the time after a serious error has occurred. And many, many errors occur: over one million adverse *preventable* events happen in hospitals in the United States every year as a result of health-care. More people die annually from accidental medical errors than from motor vehicle accidents, breast cancer, or AIDS.

> The problem to be fixed is not necessarily these honest mistakes—for "to err is human," and doctors should be allowed fallibility as equally as anyone. The problem is that a medical culture that looks away from error is a culture that can't bear to look at something as erroneously handled as congenital CMV.

I think of what Atul Gawande would make of my OB responding to me that he didn't want to worry women, rather than stopping to consider any changes he could make to prevent the next patient from sharing my fate. "For a clinician," Dr. Gawande writes, "nothing is more threatening to who you think you are than a patient with a problem you cannot solve."

"What did you expect?" Luke asks when he gets home that night, and at the look on my face, he's already backpedaling. "I'm not trying to be a jerk. I mean it literally: What did you expect? Were you hoping your doctor would say *I'm sorry?* Because, you know, doctors don't usually do that—they'll get sued if they do."

I know he's right. And yet I wanted it anyway.

———

I am not alone. Ghanaian doctor Ama Edwin, who has written about—and championed—medical truth-telling extensively, recounts that poor communication is often more of a factor in patient dissatisfaction than a doctor's negligence itself. "My experience," she writes, "has been that close to half of malpractice cases could have been avoided through disclosure or apology but instead were relegated to litigation. What the majority of patients really wanted was simply an honest explanation of what happened, and if appropriate, an apology."

One of Luke's fishing clients is a lawyer who has been coming to Sitka for twenty years to catch salmon and bring it back to his family. Over beers one evening at the Westmark Hotel, while Zaley is alternately coloring at the table and trying to sneak into the TV lounge to poke the antique bear trap, he listens to my recent research about CMV.

He's smart and savvy. One of his eyebrows is raised, the other is creased. He's not skeptical exactly, but I know he's going to push me to consider what I'm suggesting.

When I get to the part about counseling all women about CMV, he says, "Obstetricians are one of the most highly sued groups in medicine," which I didn't actually know. "And so," he explains, "discussing CMV could sink the entire industry."

"How so?" I ask.

"Well, because of how often they're sued, a private-practice obstetrical office has to make ends meet by seeing a certain number of patients every day," he explains. "So when you add a ten-minute discussion about something like CMV to every prenatal appointment, you decrease the number of women you can see in a day. Thus, you decrease your clinic's income and its ability to grow and thrive."

"So what you're saying," I suggest, "is that the CMV discussion isn't so much a burden on women as a burden on doctors themselves?"

He smiles, takes a sip of his beer. He says, "You're going to need a good lawyer."

———

I know my OB is just one doctor, and I've had only that one conversation with him. But I wonder how many other OBs are keeping CMV quiet out of ignorance or intention, despite women's desire—and right—to be informed?

After searching online for CMV experts, I find a pediatric infectious disease doctor at Baylor College of Medicine in Houston named Dr. Gail Demmler-Harrison. I call the number listed, and she answers right away—a rarity in a medical system governed by gatekeeping where I've always had to go through answering services, receptionists, nurses, machines.

I tell her briefly about Anna. Then I ask her if most OBs, not just mine, are upholding ACOG's recommendation of silence. "The paternalistic attitude of ACOG and OBs has been pervasive," she says. "Most OBs I know say that if they aren't forced to counsel women about CMV, they won't."

When I search online for a study to put numbers to Dr. Gail's experience, I find one conducted in 2007 by the CDC. I'm surprised to find that prior to 2015, ACOG actually *did* recommend that OBs discuss CMV with women. But this didn't seem to make much difference: in the 2007 CDC study, even though 90 percent of obstetricians knew that extra attention to handwashing while pregnant can reduce the risk of contracting CMV, only 44 percent counseled women on how to prevent CMV. On top of that, only 55 percent knew that avoiding children's saliva reduces the risk of contracting the disease. And less than a third of them brought up the risk of CMV-infected articles in the home—like pacifiers that have fallen to the floor, which many mothers rinse in their own mouths.

The study includes such an obvious statement, I think about calling my doctor right back: "Good hand hygiene is inexpensive, and the cost savings from preventing even one case of congenital CMV disease is high."

While I don't believe in stamping a price on the life of any child, I'm curious what the number is. When I look it up, I'm blown away: the estimated lifetime cost—including medications, hospital stays, and long-term therapies—of a single child with congenital CMV is $1.3 million. As I continue reading, another fact jars me just as equally: only 2 to 3 infants per every 10,000 have CMV as a diagnosis code in healthcare administrative data, which is one-twentieth the prevalence of CMV. This is an abysmal fail—a 5 percent if you were to grade this as though it were a test of our medical system.

The last thing I read is that the medical cost of all children with congenital CMV, in the United States alone, is somewhere between $1.9 and $4 billion per year. The range is so vast because, like all the other studies I've read about CMV, the authors suggest that more research must be done—and more babies must be tested for the disease—to accurately capture the long-term outcomes and costs of the children it affects.

But to fill larger studies requires extensive funding. And for CMV researchers to be awarded that money, medical committees first need to decide that CMV is an urgent problem to be fixed.

———

One summer in Alaska, before I had kids, I learned firsthand how decision making happens—or doesn't—even in groups of experts. I'd taken on a freelance writing assignment to travel to a remote neighboring landmass called Chichagof Island, and the pitch seemed easy enough: I'd be accompanying three scientists and a radio reporter on a mission to do "groundtruthing"—which means they'd be covering ground for days at a time to keep track of everything they saw, from native plants to invasive species to any signs humans had left behind. The goal of groundtruthing is to protect what's living by slowing down and witnessing what it is.

And Chichagof is true wilderness. There are no occupants, you can't stay there permanently, and you can't use any motors in the woods. To get there, we took a five-seater floatplane from town, flew over the tops of mountains, and landed with a series of thumps on a high-altitude lake nestled between the peaks. When the pilot flew away, we walked through the water, carrying our things above our heads. A few paces later we reached an A-frame cabin maintained by the Forest Service not far from the shore, where we set up our sleeping areas and repacked our bags with rationed food. Then we set out to log the life we saw.

We started out hiking lightly under the forest's thick canopy, plucking mushrooms for dinner, sitting down by streams to drink. But pretty soon we weren't hiking; we were bushwhacking, and it was grueling—no trails, just miles of thorny vegetation, and false summit after false summit, each rise in elevation harder than the last. I was surprised by how difficult it was, since I was the youngest and in fairly good shape. I was surprised by how far we kept going, even though the weather on the ABC Islands (Admiralty, Baranof, and Chichagof) can change without warning.

That first day, after six hours of slashing our way through and above the rainforest, we ended up on a treeless peak. Above the tundra line, Southeast Alaska spread before us in a collage of colors: jagged emerald islands cut through by teal streams, valley-size snowdrifts radiating with the magical blue of glacial ice. We stood with our hands on our hips, then sat down and stared, exhausted and in awe.

But beyond the beauty, a storm was stacking up against a ridge in the distance. I had never seen a storm like this in Southeast—black flashing cumulonimbus clouds that moved swiftly in our direction. We sat down as the darkness increased, ate bagels and M&Ms from our packs. Then in an instant, the air blew cold, and the clouds began to leak.

No one spoke. I was not just the youngest of everyone on the trip but also the least experienced in the wilderness, and when I looked around, afraid, I couldn't see anyone else's eyes to see if they were, too. Their hair was in pieces, covering their faces, and whipping in the blare of the wind. People dug through their bags for waterproof layers, but no one stood up. They zipped their jackets, tightened their shoelaces, and looked in the direction opposite the cabin, as though we'd go on. Inside, I was beginning to panic. When was someone going to say, *It's time to go back*?

Eventually, the quietest person on the trip—a biologist named

Scott—did. And then we ran. We slid downhill on any game trail we could find, belayed down the side of the mountain holding on to willow branches and hoping we'd catch roots that would hold firm where they grew sideways out of rocks. We did make it back to the cabin hours later, bleeding and drenched and happily relieved, but I felt it was foolish for us to stay out that long, to risk our lives where our radios didn't even work.

That night, sitting around the campfire, I voiced that this was how I felt because I didn't want it to happen again the next day. I wanted to make it back to Luke, to sit at Kelly's restaurant with dry hair and dry clothes and eat a sloppy burger and have the chance to appreciate life better since I hadn't died out there. And when I did—when I said to the group that we should have come back in sooner—I was surprised to find that other people felt the same.

Scott, who had worked for NOLS—the National Outdoor Leadership School—then explained something called the Abilene Complex: how sometimes, when there's a group of people, each person depends upon someone else to verbalize when the group has reached its limit or gone the wrong way and they need to reassess. When no one speaks, the group keeps going, moves beyond its boundaries, increasing their risk of danger and death.

I recognize the Abilene Complex in many situations and industries now that I know what it is. Sometimes I wonder if Luke and I might have a bit of an Abilene Complex in our marriage—if either of us will ever say about Luke's fishing for a living that we've reached as much imbalance and annual adjustment as our family can handle.

And now that we have Anna, I wonder about the Abilene Complex in medicine—how far doctors will go before one of them says, *Stop! We need to turn around. We've missed something, and we need to go back.*

3

When Anna is three weeks old and it's mid-July, my dad arrives. The quietest of men, he brings a peaceful acceptance of life to our home. Where my mom's anxiety sometimes increases my own, my dad's lack of needs puts me at ease. He could draw pictures or read books to kids all day long. He eats meals twice as slowly as anyone in our family. Growing up, I could probably count on one hand the times he raised his voice. He can play a song on the organ they have in their living room after hearing it once, and he has a childlike way about him that magnetizes kids.

Despite the shitshow that has become this summer, my dad insists that we do something fun—and when my dad insists on something, because he so rarely does, you do what he says. "I found a whale-watching cruise," he tells my mom, who fears all forms of transportation. "I think we should go."

So we do. It's a two-story boat with a biologist on board who has a long blond braid plaited over one shoulder, which is a 100 percent win for Zaley. She is riveted by female beauty, doesn't care so much about seeing animals as about watching this knowledgeable woman who cautions, "We'll hope for the best, but we might not see any whales."

We don't. We see a cinnamon-colored bear in a cove. We sneak up on a raft of sea otters, floating on their backs, the lumps of small pups on their bellies. We see yellow-beaked eagles, the forlorn faces of puffins (my favorite), the sweet pleading eyes and shiny forehead of a seal. Anna lies on the bench, contemplative and content, her skinny legs unbent, like the legs of a *Sesame Street* character—straight down, no curves.

But on the way back to town, in a trough of slight gray swells, the captain cuts the engine. The fair maiden clicks the microphone back on and, in a hush that gets everyone's immediate attention, announces: "There's a pod of orca whales right here. Everyone just wait."

Then it's like Sea World. They are poking their black and white faces out of the water and shaking their pointy noses to and fro. When they've gotten every passenger to peer over the starboard side of the boat, the whales then torpedo underneath it and come up on the port side where every passenger has now sprinted to get a glimpse. A few of them breach, then dive back down to surprise us wherever they emerge. I'm in my familiar position again—nursing Anna and rushing after Zaley with my shirt halfway up, making sure she doesn't trip and hit her head. My dad is in full-blown video mode, unable to stop collecting footage of the spectacle. Eventually, because the captain has to stay on schedule, he turns the engines back on, and we glide back toward town with six orcas escorting us at the bow of the boat, their backs rolling out of the water and back in, like some mythical beast that knows the way home.

Later, other people in town will post pictures of orcas they've seen that summer online. Never before have orcas been so prevalent in Sitka, and a biologist reports that the whales' diet indicates the species is no longer a transient population; they've decided this is where they belong.

———

While my dad plays the piano with Zaley and my mom folds the mountains of laundry that accumulate during fishing season, I drive Anna to SEARHC hospital again. It's not spelled wrong, though it still looks incorrect to me on every sign; it stands for the Southeast Alaska Regional Health Consortium. Deservedly, if you're Native Alaskan—Tlingit, Haida, Yup'ik, Inuit—everything here is covered for free. But as non-Natives, we will pay for all our care, and when I walk past the reception desk, I can feel the bills being processed, the financial impact of our mere entry into the building. It's our tenth visit in one week. And it's a big one: this time I'll be having a look at my child's brain.

I take the elevator to the second floor, to radiology, the reality of which makes my brain flicker momentarily. I enter a dark room where the ultrasound tech is waiting. As soon as I tell her the name of Anna's disease, she exclaims, "My daughter has CMV!"

My pulse rockets up. But quickly I realize she misunderstands. "Yeah," she says, "she had all those viruses in her teens: CMV, mononucleosis, Epstein-Barr. We couldn't figure out what was going on. She was tired for months."

"Congenital CMV is a little different," I tell her, trying for gentle, not corrective. "I caught it while I was pregnant. I'm here to see if my daughter has brain damage."

"Oh." Silence spreads its heavy curtain over the room. She readies a computer that looks like the first one my dad bought in the early 1990s, with a flashing white cursor on a square black screen. "The good thing," she says, aiming for connection again, "is that babies' heads were practically designed for ultrasounds. The soft spot is a perfect opening to look into their brain."

She pats the paper sheet on the exam table, indicating it's where I should sit. So I do, laying Anna down next to me in her heather-pink, button-down onesie.

"Now, I've never used this machine on a newborn before. And it's probably thirty years old," she says, slathering Anna's fontanelle with ultrasound goo. "But let's just see what we see."

Despite her pleasantness, this feels worse than the hearing test. The dread is not just nauseating but cold. The window is open, and like so many windows in Sitka, it should be closed. When the wet breeze blows in, the daylight flaps rudely into the room. In my jacket, I shiver. Anna looks up at me with eyes that don't yet know words or judgments, just pictures. Her world is me; I am her one picture. How I wish, some days, that we could just look at each other, oblivious, forever. I'm afraid to know the state of her brain. It almost feels like a violation, this peering in and making predictions—and predictions, I now know, are total illusions when it comes to the spontaneous and idiosyncratic development of children.

What I'm afraid of is me. I don't want what I see to alter my perception of Anna's future—which could, actually, affect her future. If Anna has calcifications—chunky bright spots on imaging, which occur in 70 percent of CMV infants who are symptomatic at birth and can indicate developmental challenges —will I treat her as though she's already delayed? If I see the ghostly specters of white matter disease in her brain—which can be a sign of seizures to come—will I be on constant watch, disallowing her a natural zone-out, a twitch, a whole night of sleep?

The human brain has 86 billion neurons, a number I can't conceive of in the least. On top of this, each neuron can have up to fifteen thousand connections with other neurons via synapses. How is it, I wonder, that a single picture of Anna's brain could tell us anything about her constellation-size immensity? I think of Psalm 139, which my dad had inscribed for me, after Zaley was born, in his perfect wedding-invitation calligraphy, and which sits in a dark teal frame in her room at home: "For you created my inmost being; you knit me together in my mother's womb. I praise you because I am fearfully and wonderfully made."

I steel myself with an image of these lines before the ultrasound machine looks inside. Anna does have an inmost being and an immensity of connection-making brain matter—an intricate mind and an invisible soul all her own—no matter what I'm about to see.

The tech gently places the wand on Anna's fontanelle. On the screen, there's a circular black orb with white speckles, and a little wormlike thing that pulsates—which the sonographer says is blood pumping through a coil. The tech swishes around inside Anna's head, her professional silence a comfort and an alarm.

"So," she finally says, pausing in an aerial view of the amazing, mushy entity inside my daughter that will control her everything. "All I can tell is that her ventricles are larger on one side than the other," which I know can indicate a condition associated with CMV called ventriculomegaly, which, like all sequelae of CMV, can mean absolutely nothing or can mean future disability. "But again, this machine is probably older than you. And asymmetrical ventricles might be the case inside your brain or mine, we've just never looked at ours up close.

"I'm no radiologist," she concludes, "but the rest of it looks clear."

That evening, because the phrase *it looks clear* is a triumphant refrain in my head, we decide to meet up with friends. We drive out to the end of the road and park at the trailhead to Mosquito Cove, where you can see the ferry terminal and all the green and yellow freight containers that bring furniture and electronics, food and vehicles to the island. A stone's throw from the coast, my friend Lisa is leaning over a firepit, turning a squat cast iron kettle on a crank. When I sit down in a camping chair close by, the pot begins to explode with crackles, then clumps of popcorn. "Of all the things I've owned in Alaska," she says, grinning and pulling it expertly off the fire with a glove, "this one is my favorite."

Lisa delivered a stillborn baby in Sitka. They moved away after that, unable to bear the pain this location kept placing before them. Then a few years later, she and her husband, Pete, a Coast Guard pilot, put in a request to come back. They've spent eight total years here, and now they have six kids they're raising in Sitka. Whenever I'm struggling with the coming and going of our seasons here, I think of Lisa's willingness to start over every four years. She says she does it because God always provides the women she needs.

The rain is lifting now, the same way it came, in wispy curtains that go up now instead of down. Anna is asleep and warm in my lap, Luke and Pete are on the beach drinking Rainiers, and Zaley is giggling at Lisa's boys, who have waded out, waist-high, into the stripes of dark blue water. The evenings here are such a salve for the days. The weather seems to open up this time of night, just like the energy in our homes, once the dads are finished working and the rain has rained enough.

Every few seconds a humpy salmon leaps skyward from the surface, wiggles in the air, and flops back in. Luke says no one knows why salmon and whales breach like this, flinging their bodies, crescent-shaped, from their environment. Some say it's an attempt at parasite removal or communication. Each time a fish blasts up, the kids shriek with delight. I never tire of watching them fly. It doesn't seem random or pained. It looks like an act of celebration to me.

4

When it's time to get Anna's drugs, I brace myself, then dial the number of our insurance company.

We have a history. Initially, they decided that I never gave birth to Anna, therefore they wouldn't cover the cost of her delivery.

"Authorizations," I say into the phone, but I have to say it three times because Zaley's voice near the receiver is scrambling up mine. Whoever invented automated voice answering services didn't have kids in the background in mind. "I need authorizations"—now I am yelling—"for a medication for my daughter."

It must be that my volume or anger quotient trips something in their system, because then a real live human gets on the line. "Okay," she says, chirpy. "Can you please tell me the name of the medication?"

"The drug is called valganciclovir," I say. "My daughter has a disease called congenital CMV."

"Can you say that last part again?"

"C as in Cat. M as in Mary. V as in Victor."

"CMV," she says. "I've never heard of it. And it's not in our system. Can you please hold?"

An hour later, she gets back on the line to tell me it's not looking like they'll approve coverage of Anna's antiviral, which will cost $900 a month. I'll have to pursue self-pay.

Luckily, I'm distracted from insurance rage because there's a knock on the door. On the wet deck is a thin package from London. When Zaley rips it open, she's disappointed, and I'm thrilled: it's *Stealth Virus*, Dr. Paul Griffiths's book about CMV. I start reading the book before I've even sat down, and right away I see that maybe CMV's shortcomings began in the beginning, when it first received its name.

Dr. Griffiths explains that CMV was originally given its acronym and brought to public attention in 1957 by Thomas Weller and John Enders, the same two Nobel Prize–winning scientists who'd grown measles, rubella, polio, and varicella (chicken pox) at their Harvard University lab—and who would later help to eliminate all the diseases they studied except for CMV. Weller, a father of four who was interested in natural history and fish, was in his lab growing CMV from disabled babies when he noticed that under a microscope, many of their cells looked similar and odd. They were owl-eyed and huge, thus the breakdown of the name he would devise: *mega* means "gigantic" and *cyto* means "cells."

Saying *CMV* aloud, I hear its dissonance, its lack of music. It's such a tightly bound acronym, short, with no vowels, and its long-form doesn't help; *cytomegalovirus* sounds more like a dinosaur than a disease—clunky, lumbering, and like it must be obsolete.

While the naming of CMV was certainly an important milestone, I wish Weller had given Anna's disease a more memorable label like *measles* or *polio*—or a sexier name, like *Zika* will earn the summer Anna turns one. All these names you can pronounce as words, not as three letters that clang against each other and then roll right out of a person's head. Almost every time I tell someone what Anna has, they ask me what it stands for, then they ask me to say it again.

Dr. Griffiths writes that even though CMV had already been around for hundreds of millions of years, until Thomas Weller came along, it hadn't yet been pinpointed as a commonality in children who had intellectual or physical delays. Neither had anyone associated the fluids of young children with any kind of risk until Weller recovered CMV samples from living children with CMV—as opposed to by autopsy—and realized that they continued to excrete the virus for many months. Weller recognized that the infection could spread rapidly in groups of preschool children, whether they had congenital CMV or not. He rightly saw the danger of CMV during pregnancy as an urgent issue in the realm of public health.

But what is public health? I've learned since having Anna: a primary care doctor or specialist tends to treat people who are sick, whereas public health agencies and physicians aim to *prevent* groups of people from ever getting sick in the first place. They do this, primarily, through research, education of the public, and the administration of available vaccines. According to the American Public Health Association's language online: "Public health saves money, improves our quality of life, helps children thrive and reduces human suffering."

What I notice when I read this mission statement—besides the priority of prevention—is the plural forms of its nouns: public health is about *children,* not one child; it's about collective human suffering, not the treatments we choose for ourselves.

Which is why, I realize, all the studies I've been reading about women's desires to know or not know about CMV are inherently flawed. This shouldn't be about what each woman wants. What an embarrassingly short-sighted way to think about a much farther-reaching problem.

What about CMV everywhere else? I read online that in sub-Saharan Africa (where CMV infection is widespread in the general population), when mothers have both HIV and CMV in their serum at delivery, the women have a tenfold increase in maternal death (CMV worsens the effects of HIV) and a fourfold increase in the mortality of their HIV-infected infants by the age of two.

In another article I find, Dr. Tatiana Lanzieri, a medical epidemiologist who researches CMV in other resource-limited countries where people have high birth rates, live in close proximity, and tend to watch each other's children, writes: "The aggregate number of children born with congenital CMV infection is likely to be enormous."

When I email Dr. Suresh Boppana, an infectious disease specialist in Alabama who has authored many of the international CMV studies I've read, I ask him what exactly *enormous* means. He emails me back promptly with numbers based on birth rates for each country and available CMV data—which is, predictably, lacking. Nonetheless, the numbers are staggering: in Nigeria, between 65,000 and 130,000 children are born annually with congenital CMV. In India, up to 540,000 babies are born every year with the disease.

And the children who are symptomatic have far worse outcomes than they do here. They don't get referrals to audiology and neurology and infectious disease. Early Intervention doesn't knock on the door with resistance bands and medicine balls and flash cards. Deaf advocacy organizations don't call the parents, and the child's providers are not connected through a sophisticated digital database system. Parents cannot seek out centers for the blind, autism programs, or private therapies that target eating problems or vestibular dysfunction.

Children who are deaf won't likely get hearing aids or cochlear implants or sign language instruction. Children with gross motor delays won't be fitted for power wheelchairs or walkers or braces. What they are more likely to get is neglect, abuse, or total abandonment.

A friend of mine from New Orleans who adopted two children—one with spina bifida and one with Down syndrome—from an orphanage in Ukraine says the system is full of children with congenital CMV. The thought of Anna, left on a threadbare mattress, in a room with twenty other crying atypical kids, nearly makes me sick.

To say that CMV might worry women here is to lack the imagination for a world beyond our own convenience. To say that CMV is too difficult a discussion denies the existence of millions of children suffering in less developed places. It also impedes these children from the dignity of a diagnosis and timely treatment.

I think back to when I first read the words *global public health crisis* and how the phrase felt too powerful for me to understand. Now I get it. The crisis is not the children; the crisis is that we aren't talking about a way to save them.

Besides our failure to recognize CMV's impact on a global scale, Dr. Paul Griffiths explains in *Stealth Virus* another problem with CMV: in the 1950s, while Thomas Weller was bent over his microscope, slowly trying to understand the complexities of CMV, other doctors were doing the opposite, drawing hasty conclusions from a more simplified, inauthentic version of CMV. They were using a cultured strain of CMV, meaning it had evolved in a lab, and it turns out, this strain had lost eighteen genes found in the wild, unattenuated virus—the living one that infects human beings.

Because the cultured version of CMV did not respond well to researchers' attempts to create a vaccine, the majority of doctors and researchers wrote CMV off as a futile project, with no hope for eradication.

Thomas Weller feared the fallout from this flawed work, which was published in prominent medical journals. He cautioned against using the insufficient strains being traded between labs. And foreseeing a world where CMV continued to stealthily disable kids, he remained adamant that CMV not be buried by layers of misconception and ignorance. There could be little doubt, he wrote, in his landmark CMV article in the *New England Journal of Medicine* in 1971, that CMV had a greater toll than rubella in terms of personal tragedy and economic loss.

But rubella had things going for it that CMV has never had: rubella tends to occur in acute bursts, during seasonal epidemics, and it presents in women with a visible rash. Whereas, Griffiths writes, "CMV silently infected women year in, year out; they could not seek advice because they were not aware that they had a problem."

Thomas Weller was among a dedicated handful of others, including Dr. Griffiths, who not only recognized the silent presentation of CMV but also knew that Western medicine was leaving an important disease behind. But even when Dr. Griffiths aimed to publish some of the new findings about CMV (such as the fact that women who'd already had it were not fully immune and could catch it again), his scientific evidence drew renewed skepticism. Where data should have ruled, it was trumped by prevailing medical opinion.

In *Stealth Virus,* though—which I bring to the beach and to playgrounds and to coffeeshops, reading a paragraph at a time while Zaley is briefly distracted by abalone shells or friends—I keep track of the litany of scientists and researchers who still have not written off CMV. Every time Dr. Griffiths mentions a doctor I haven't heard of, I pull a sand-crusted notebook out of my diaper bag and jot down the name: Martha Yow, Pablo Sanchez, Suresh Boppana, Michael Cannon, Karen Fowler, Mark Schleiss—most of whom, like Dr. Griffiths himself, are devoting their lives, against the medical mainstream, to the problem of my daughter's disease.

Each night I pick one of these doctors and read his or her studies in medical journals online. The most outspoken author I find is
a doctor named Mike Cannon, an epidemiologist at the CDC and
one of only two people assigned to CMV at the agency, who wrote
an article called "Washing Our Hands of the Congenital Cytomegalovirus Disease Epidemic." In it, he echoes Thomas Weller when he
writes: "Perhaps no single cause of birth defects and developmental
disabilities in the United States currently provides greater opportunity for improved outcomes in more children than congenital CMV."
And to my great appreciation: "Given the present state of knowledge,
women deserve to be informed."

But when I look at the publication date, my gut goes concave.
His outcry to educate more doctors and women about CMV was
published in 2005, a decade earlier. And here I am, a mother who'd
never heard of CMV, whirlpooling through a cycle of research and
confusion and trying to convince the medical system not only that
my newborn needs rapid treatment, but that her virus even exists.

When the insurance lady says she can't find CMV and won't
approve its treatment, I'm beginning to understand that I'm fighting
nearly a century of misconceptions, which have resulted in countless articles and lists—at OBs offices, at hospital nurseries, at health
insurance companies—that all lack the letters C-M-V.

5

I take to calling insurance repeatedly, in quick succession, to see if I can reach someone with a nicer voice than the prior person. But each representative insists that we haven't exhausted other treatment possibilities—even though there aren't any. There's just this one drug that will stop any damage to my daughter's *brain,* which I enunciate emphatically, impressing on them the vulnerability of my daughter's one functioning mind.

I ask for letters from both pediatricians, which they both draft immediately, but because I also need the drug immediately and I need to be a mother to my children—not on the phone incessantly—we will end up paying for valgancyclovir out of pocket.

Now I need a pharmacist. And not just any pharmacist—I need a saint. I am looking for a total stranger, in Juneau, who will arrange for a pilot and transport the antiviral from the pharmacy to the airport tarmac as soon as it arrives. They will also need to notify me of the flight's ETA so I can receive the medicine as soon as it touches down, lest its temperature rise or fall. I feel like James Bond, minus the cool car and jawline and know-how.

I picture the Walgreens in Denver, five minutes from our house, and the luxury of pulling up to the drive-through with kids in seatbelts to magically retrieve any medicine we need. I'm sick for home, feel sick toward Alaska—its pointless isolation and outdated systems, its fickle weather and stupid distance. I wonder, for the hundredth time, why anyone would ever have settled here in the first place.

———

Because Luke chose Alaska, it's an entirely different animal for him.

And because I'll never make the ultimatum that many fishing mothers I know have made—*it's Alaska or us*—he can also choose when we're finished living here. This is an argument we have every summer: what are the limits of motherhood, and when do you know you've reached them, other than when you've already exceeded them? What he does is a grind for him, too, but it's a grind with purpose and two horsepower engines and reasonable adults in his space all day long, while I'm stranded on a narrow strip of land, with a car I'm afraid to drive, trying to reason with little people who lack a prefrontal cortex, logic, and all self-control.

Luke was also born with a work ethic coursing through his blood. His dad, Willis, was born on a dairy farm, the youngest of seven kids, and there was no reprieve for the baby of the family; it was up early, milk the Holsteins, feed the needy calves. An award-winning leader and businessman today, Willis's motto is "Never had a bad day in my life." And he means it. In a similar way, a hard day for Luke is a good day, whereas a hard day for me is self-annihilating. After the last ten years of crying to Luke about how difficult this lifestyle can be for me, I'm coming to see that his main issue—possibly his only issue—with Alaska is me.

But if it is, he never says the things to me that he could, like *get it together* or *shape up*. Pacifist that he is, he apologizes for how hard it must be. He tells me what a good job I'm doing (to which I, through tears, guffaw). He is what I am not: calm. At the Orthodox church, where we go to vespers on Saturday evenings, after I give up on medical phone calls for the week, he puts his first two fingers and thumb together and makes the sign of the cross as he kisses an icon of Saint Herman, his favorite saint, who happens to be a lifelong transplant to this state.

In fact, I think if Luke hadn't married me, he might have become a modern-day monastic, a second Saint Herman—a gentle, unflappable man who slept on a bench on a deerskin hide, moved from Kodiak to the much more isolated Spruce Island, where he pursued a life of solitude but was found by followers because he was good at settling disputes and unafraid of illness, even an epidemic that impacted his closest friends, the native Aleuts. When asked how he could tolerate a life largely alone in the woods, he said, "I am not alone. God is here, as God is everywhere."

This is, essentially, what Luke chants at vespers and at home some evenings, with Zaley at his side learning the harmony. "Oh Heavenly King, the Comforter, the Spirit of Truth," they sing, "Who art everywhere present and fillest all things. Come and abide in us, and cleanse us from every impurity." Oh, how I wish I could have Luke's outlook and remember the healing capacity of these lines—the spirit of goodness, the comfort we can find in every earthbound thing.

But in my life, it's a constant struggle to not let goodness and depth get edged out by daily frustrations and logistics. And as soon as I have to call insurance, I forget that God exists.

Maybe this is why I like going to church this summer more than usual: here I can't get anything done, can't make those calls, and I feel closer to my family, to silence, to peace. I stare at the brown beeswax candles flickering in tall stands of sand. I listen to the light taps of rain on the thin French windows. On the left of the altar, underneath a suspended lantern, is a miraculous icon of Mary. People come from all over the world to pray at the foot of this icon, asking for Mary's intercession, and many believe her gaze has restored their poor health. The icon is silver-plated, and she is holding her golden-robed infant. Her eyes are demanding, intense. It's hard to look away, hard to say why she both comforts and provokes. It's because, I suppose, she's a mother who knows the utter power and the unbearable vulnerability of her child.

———

Not knowing where to start, and not actually feeling like James Bond at all, I simply call the first pharmacy listed online for the city of Juneau. The person who answers the phone is the manager, and his name is Michael. I explain our predicament and my desperation to get the drug within forty-eight hours: Anna is three and a half weeks old and she needs to start it before she's four weeks of age. "Let me work on this," Michael says. "But I promise I'll do everything I can."

I believe him. Most people don't use the word *promise* lightly, especially when they're promising something to a mother who sounds like me.

While I make lunch, clean the kitchen counter, feed the baby, draw an erupting volcano, and try to find a snack with less than twenty grams of sugar that Zaley will eat, Michael is spending the same afternoon finding a pharmacy in the Lower 48 that will ship the prescription to him in the right temperature-safe packaging. Then he is figuring out the flight schedules for every small plane that will fly from Juneau to Sitka. And then he makes a phone call to me, telling me he has found a pharmacy down south and a pilot up here, who will hopefully make our convoluted scheme a reality.

The specialty pharmacy in Indiana calls me next for my information. They're readying the package for Juneau the following morning.

———

The next day is a toilet bowl of rain. Whenever it wanes, Zaley and I scurry out to the deck. She draws a giant chalk *X* in pink, as though the plane might drop the package at our feet. "When will it land, Mama?" she asks. "In the next six days? The next six hours? The next six minutes?" She has a thing for six. "Hopefully by six o'clock, sweetie," but I desperately hope not, because by then, the charter planes might be finished for the day, given what one Raven Radio host has just called "a river in the sky."

My phone rings. It's Michael.

"The medicine is in Juneau," he says. "But it isn't on the plane."

I sit down on the ground, crushed.

"When I opened the package to double-check that it was correct," he tells me, "I noticed it had been sent in powder form, not liquid."

"What does that mean?" I ask, almost frantic.

"It's actually fine. It means you don't have to rush it home. It will be the right temperature whenever you mix it. I just needed to write you some instructions for how to reconstitute it," he says, bubbly now. But I swear, he sounds a little short of breath.

"Is everything okay?" I ask.

"Yes," he says. "It's just . . . I'm on my way to the airport with it now."

Knowing he's the manager of the pharmacy, I ask, "You're *personally* driving it there?"

And he says, "No. I'm walking. Actually . . . I'm running!"

The rain has turned monsoon heavy, so I suit up the girls in their head-to-toe raingear, which takes about the same amount of time as the flight from Juneau to Sitka: twenty-two minutes. Then I speed to the airport in the non-defrosting Suburban, swiping a quarter of the gigantic windshield with my hand when I can't see the road. I park as close as I can to the door, and the three of us shuffle inside to the windows at the back of the airport, just in time to see a pilot running down the slick metal stairs outside his shining plane. In his hands is the white Styrofoam box I've been picturing, just as I've pictured it. Inside is Anna's tutti-frutti-flavored medicine that we'll give her twice a day for the next six months.

We meet the pilot in the doorway, on the dry side of a waterfall of rain. Zaley reaches for the box with both arms outstretched. He looks at me for consent, and after I nod, he gently hands it to her. When I try to thank him, I am cry-inhaling too hard, so Zaley says it for me: "Kanks you so much."

I stand at the kitchen sink, read Michael's note, and tear up again. The syringe is the tiniest one I have ever seen, its width the size of a child's birthday candle. I add water to the powder and watch the cloud of elements combine. It feels powerful, this vial, like a serum given to a hero in need. I know it's unlikely that the medicine will restore Anna's hearing, if she has any, but I also know it might stop CMV—and this is my mission. I give the bottle a few shakes, pull the liquid into the skinny syringe, and slide it against Anna's inner cheek. Her eyes zero in on mine as she swallows every drop.

Jerry, at the lab, is back from vacation. And even though he's a large, big-handed man, he gets Anna's vein every time. He's also gentle and kind to me, knowing how much her pain triggers mine. Her numbers are staying level, which means she's tolerating this one chance to treat the trespass of her disease.

But one morning, after the grief of my parents leaving, Dr. Vastola calls. We need to talk. And we need to talk to someone else: Shannon Hughes is the PA (physician assistant) who manages the infectious disease department's CMV clinic at Children's Hospital Colorado, and together we should have a conference call to make sure we're doing everything we need to do.

On the morning of the call, I go to the mothers' Rosary group at the Catholic church, then I buckle the kids into the car, but I don't drive anywhere. I climb into the back, squashing myself between my daughters—I have no childcare, and nowhere better to restrain my kids.

Shannon is a wealth of knowledge—more so than anyone I've spoken to about CMV. She has an impressive grasp of its epidemiology, contagiousness, medications, and statistics, and the call is going fairly smoothly because any time Zaley interrupts, I pop an M&M into her mouth. But Shannon can't tell me anything about Anna's potential outcomes. "The upside," she said, "is you're already doing everything you could be doing, which is the antiviral Anna's already taking."

This makes me feel good and terrible: yes, she's on the drug, despite the complications of obtaining it. But really, is there nothing else we could be doing, if we're to give Anna every chance any other child would have?

Both providers agree that we can wait until late September to address Anna's hearing and vision since no providers in town can do so. Shannon goes on to say that assistive devices like hearing aids or glasses are not so time-sensitive that a few months' delay will impede Anna's progress.

But once the conference call ends and I call Somer—the audiologist in town whom we'd seen briefly the week prior—she strongly disagrees with the choice we've made for me to stay. "You should have included me in the conversation," she says sternly. "I've spoken to audiologists at the children's hospitals in Denver and Seattle, and we believe it's imperative you have Anna's hearing checked soon."

"What do you mean *soon*?" I ask.

"I mean, like, next week."

If we don't get Anna fitted for hearing aids now, we'll be delaying the six-month process of candidacy for cochlear implants, if she is, in fact, completely deaf. I don't even know what cochlear implants are. But I take what Somer says next very seriously: two months of delay at such an early age could impact Anna's language development noticeably.

This I feel with ice-cold certainty: to take away communication would be to take away everything. Somer suggests we fly to Seattle, where she can set up a team of specialists to receive us as soon as we arrive.

———

I need to talk to Luke. I ask my friend Jules if she'll come over and watch Zaley when our husbands are done fishing that evening. Jules has two kids who are ten and twelve, named Johnny and Emma, and to Zaley, these kids are Sitka's sun and moon. When they arrive, Zaley's whole body shakes with excitement, and she doesn't even hear me when I say goodbye.

I put Anna in the back of the car, hoping she'll sleep, and by the time I reach Jefferson Davis Street and the house without a dryer where we once lived, I can hear the rhythm of her breath. Then I pull into the harbor to pick up Luke.

I love to watch him walk up the ramp from his boat—his metal coffee thermos swinging at this side, his big running legs slow but still springy when walking on land. He smiles when he sees me in the two-hour parking lot, and gets in.

"I thought we'd go for a drive," I say.

He nods. He can see I'm about to cry, so he takes my hand strongly in his and puts it on the console between us. Without letting go of him, I drive.

On Sawmill Creek Road, we pass people sorting their boxes and cans at the recycling plant, the white crosses in the trees where the Russian cemetery is nearly overtaken by ferns, the wet green rows of giant veggies at the You-Pick Farm. After passing the cement whale spines jutting out of the sand at Whale Park, the road opens up dramatically to the expanse of Silver Bay—a spectacular junction of mountains and ocean, where purple peaks echo past each other, their silhouettes fading into a powder-white sky. A lonely waterfall trickles down Bear Mountain and into the bay where the fish hatchery releases millions of newborn salmon to replenish these waters that we borrow from so heavily.

"I need to go to Seattle," I tell him.

"Okay," he says. "We'll make it happen."

"I'm worried, Luke. Like really worried."

He's looking out the window, toward the falling water, this man who can fix a lower engine unit, a girl's braid, a good dinner—just about anything. He turns to me, not dismissive but honest, and says, "No matter what, Meg, we'll love her just the same."

———

And so I cry. I cry the whole way back, into my not-quite-waterproof raincoat and the damp, navy blue upholstery of our car. I've cried in Indian River, in the harbor's concrete restrooms, in the Pacific's already-salted waters. I plan to cry over dinner, while doing dishes, and in the shower.

But once we churn up the hill to home, spots of blue are bleeding between the clouds—"sucker holes," we call them in Alaska, because they'll trick you into believing the sun is on its way. I dry my eyes standing in our yard. I guess I am a sucker because I love the sight of those holes, the seratonin triggered by that particular nonreplicable blue, no matter if the clouds are going to close back up.

Inside, when I tell Jules we've decided I should take Anna to Seattle, she immediately offers to watch Zaley for a few days. Z can sleep in Emma's bed, eat chocolate chip pancakes when she wakes up, and take the dogs for a walk with John. So that night I book a single round-trip ticket to Seattle. Luke's mom, Anita, calls me from Colorado and offers me a gift that will be more saving than I know: she and Luke's dad are going to meet me there.

6

Seattle is busy and of a more industrial gray than Sitka from above, then warmer than I'm used to when Anna and I exit the breezeway. A futuristic train takes us between terminals, and I feel the strange orbit of some other, faster planet. It's sunny, and the brazen light feels exposing. Luke's parents are standing near the luggage claim next to two white chairs, and I realize, seeing them in their excited smiles and down-south clothes—nicer and brighter than anything you'd wear in Alaska—that I haven't seen them since the diagnosis. Hugging them, I fall apart.

We check into a hotel that overlooks Lake Union. Beyond the long window, people are jumping off their boats into a sheet of tinfoil-like water. Watching them, I feel displacement and peace. Seattle and its happy strangers offer a vague comfort: I don't have to explain anything to anyone for a brief pause in time. I can be in a place as unfamiliar as the place Anna has opened in our lives.

We walk along the water. We trade off Anna. We eat somewhere. Then it's nighttime, the sky goes unnaturally dark for this time of our year, and I realize with a rattle of dread that I've forgotten to pack the syringe for Anna's medication.

As Anita and I speed through curving black streets, newly slickened by a light nighttime rain, I can't believe this has become my life. Not only is the urban evening and its organized lamplight peculiar to me already, after only a month in small-town Alaska, so is the now-estranged carefreeness of typical lives. It's ten p.m., the time of night you'd find only closed doors and a few wayward drinkers in downtown Sitka. But in Seattle, young couples are entering and exiting trendy restaurants with geometrical wallpaper and orange outdoor chairs. Groups sip wine under awnings, have nowhere to be, aren't looking for medical supplies this time of night.

I know these people have issues in their lives, too, but it's the first time I can see that my daughter's life will be different in ways the able-bodied world doesn't seem to represent. And I know something they have yet to learn: that we're all more vulnerable than we can possibly believe—that a tiny, invisible virus can change the way you eat, think, live, and breathe.

We find a CVS, and Anita pulls over. Compared to the general store in Sitka, which closes before dinner, the CVS is bustling with people buying what seems like everything. With one sweep of my vision, I can see children's toys and scarves, lipstick and shoes, alcohol and loaves of bread. There's a bank of freezers with more ice cream than you can buy at a grocery store in Sitka. I want everything. I want nothing. Anna's single need pulses in the foreground, and everything in my periphery seems a tremendous array of excess.

The pharmacy is in the back, and I walk past all the cosmetics and lotions, snagging a Neutrogena sunscreen that's half the price it is in Alaska. I've brought Anna's medication with me, and I show the pharmacist that I need a syringe the size of the tiny hole on top. She takes the bottle from me and pops the plastic lid with the tiny hole off the top. Then she pops a new lid onto it with an accordion that expands inside the bottle so it won't leak. And then she gives me a centimeter-thick syringe with huge numbers on it denoting the dosage, that perfectly fits the new hole. With my eyes wide in adoration, I bring the plunger to an exactitude I have not yet been able to give my daughter.

"Amazing," I whisper.

"Do you want a few more to take with you?" the pharmacist asks, kindly but like I might be a little unstable.

"YES!" I say. Then I thank her three times, pay for my lotion, and reenter the twilight zone of Seattle at night. In the back seat of the car, I lean over Anna, glide the syringe into her mouth, and slowly push the exact measurement of medicine past her tongue.

———

The next morning is blazing with surrounding water and sun. Anita drives us across two long bridges to the Bellevue Seattle Children's Hospital. There's a Blue Angels airshow that weekend, and fighter jets are cartwheeling in the sky, the white tails of their exhaust double-helixed together like airborne DNA. I consider the jobs Anna won't be able to do with hearing or vision impairments, and I wonder if flying is one of them.

At the hospital, while checking us in, the receptionist asks if my baby or I have been exposed to any infectious diseases. She means Ebola, since the Ebola outbreak began in Africa a year ago, in 2014. But we are carrying a much closer, more prevalent disease. I don't know how to respond. I don't want to compromise our appointment since it was the only time before September they could see us here.

"My daughter has congenital CMV," I say.

"So . . . no?" she replies.

While I decide how to answer, the receptionist's hand floats up, then rests on the top of her abdomen. She's pregnant.

"CMV is an infectious disease," I tell her. "So yes."

She taps a few keys. "Never heard of it. Just have a seat over there till you're called."

———

Anita and I sit down on a C-shaped lime-green couch. A few minutes later two audiologists approach us in suits, and one of them says Anna's name. We follow them into a large office with high ceilings, where the familiar family of wires and a reclining chair with a few pillows awaits.

"We'll just have you sit here," one of them tells me, "And if you can nurse her to sleep, we'll begin."

I sit in the recliner, and Anita takes a smaller chair by the door. The suction cups go on Anna's head, the cords in her ears, and the clicks begin. Never at a loss for topics to discuss, Anita and I whisper about the kids, the husbands, the hunting, the fishing. The test rolls on and like girls in church, we stifle giggles about Luke and his dad's similarities—their maddening optimism, their passion for vacuuming—and we plan out the rest of the day. Toward the end of the test, Anita, who brings candy wherever she goes, offers me some licorice.

As I'm eating a Red Vine, one of the audiologists gently strips the tape from the sides of Anna's head and removes the wires from her ears. The other one rolls her chair over to me. In her hands, she holds up an audiogram—the sheet of paper that shows the levels and frequencies of what we hear, as represented by small pictograms on a chart: leaves falling, water pouring, the gentle purr of an open fridge. A baby crying, a dog barking, a lawn mower mowing. A chainsaw, a motorcycle, a jet engine roaring. The audiologist brings her hand below all the pictures and moves it from one side to the other.

The sweeping of her hand below the chart—the sweeping away of all those sounds—is a motion I'll remember forever.

"What we've found is that Anna didn't have any response in either ear," she says softly. "This indicates a profound hearing loss"—as though I should know what this means.

I set the rest of my licorice down. Take a hard swallow.

"It means she cannot hear at the limits of our equipment. She wouldn't hear a jet engine if she were standing next to it."

I'm silent, truly stunned. It seems like there's a word she's not saying, and I want an understandable definition, the clarity of her diagnosis and its connotation. I want to hear what the truth will sound like when I tell Luke, Zaley, my mom and dad, and all our family members and friends what Anna is.

"Are you telling me she's *deaf*?" I ask.

And the audiologist says, "Yes."

———

I feel I'm underwater. The audiologists' two voices become one, but it goes low and distant, and then it's like that voice makes no sound. My eyes are filling, then pouring over, and the tears are landing on Anna's neck, waking her. Someone hands me a Kleenex.

"We'll give you a minute," an audiologist says. "This is difficult news to take in."

They slip out the door like eels, and Anita slides her chair over to mine so we are knees to knees. The world feels tilted. It's quieter and louder. There is Anna, awake now, with her dark soft hair and dark soft eyes. She's the same child as always, and yet so very changed. I feel it's insensitive to make words of this moment, which feels so shattering and also so sacred, and my sobs are giant, heaving silences. Anita has one hand on my arm and one on Anna's back, and knowing I am in a place perhaps untouchable, she, too, leaves this juncture wordless, intact.

———

Then the audiologists come in the door again. While my ears and heart swell and drum, their voices are controlled and sensibly calm. There are logistics to figure out, if I can. We need to mold her ears for hearing aids (which will be ready in a few months when we return to Colorado), and I need to choose a color. *Hearing aids?* I think. *But she's deaf.* The audiologist answers before I have to ask.

"It's not likely the hearing aids will give her much information," she says. "With her level of hearing loss, she may pick up a low frequency here or there, but nothing that resembles language. The reason she'll wear these is to keep her auditory cortex stimulated. And to prove to your insurance that she's worn them reliably for six months to little effect. Then insurance is more likely to cover the cost of cochlear implants."

"Which is?"

"With the surgery and everything, probably around $400,000."

While I chew on the enormity of this sum, the other audiologist brings out a plastic board with ten hearing aids in different colors affixed to it. I know Zaley would have loved this part, and I want to pick a color she'll like. There's cobalt blue, fluorescent green, a marbled orange and red. At the bottom is a champagne-like muted rose. I choose this: just girly enough, "pretty classy," Anita says, and Zaley can still call it pink. The audiologists squeeze a bubblegum-colored goo into each of Anna's ears, then extract stiffened globs that mirror the perfect contours of her nonworking features.

"Do you want to see how cochlear implants work, in case you choose to go that route?" an audiologist asks. She already has a picture and a model poised on her lap, so I say yes.

"Unlike with hearing aids, which can only amplify sounds going through the ear, cochlear implants bypass the ear entirely and could give Anna almost full access to sound."

Had I heard her right? *Full access to sound?* This seems like miracle work, like a premature erasure of the deafness to which I've just been introduced. My vision goes a little spinny. I try to pay attention.

"Cochlear implants are designed to mimic the function of the human ear," the audiologist explains with a diagram of an ear the size of my head. "The cochlea is the part of the inner ear that converts sound waves into nerve signals, which the brain processes as hearing. The cochlea are lined with hair cells, which wiggle and detect sound. Anna's cochlea are all too damaged to work because of CMV. The idea with cochlear implants is to stimulate the follicle *underneath* each dead hair cell—mimicking the way the ear sends sounds to the brain."

She holds up a cochlear implant next. It looks like a large hearing aid. But attached to the processor that hangs on the ear is a long, thin coil that ends at a half-dollar-size disk. This disk is actually a magnet that holds on to another magnet—a magnet embedded underneath the skin.

Before CIs work, a doctor must surgically implant those internal magnets above each ear, between a patient's scalp and skull. Additionally, a gelatinous, electrode-studded strip is threaded through each inner ear, like a blade of grass being pushed through a shell. When the CI is on, sounds enter the external processor through a tiny microphone. From there, they travel up to the coil to the magnet, then cascade down the internal coil, delivering an electronic sensation of sound directly to the brain.

This all happens two weeks after a CI patient heals from surgery, when an audiologist activates the external devices—removable processors that Anna could take off any time she slept or preferred silence.

But it wasn't like she'd just hear, *bam,* like that, when we activated the implants. All sounds would begin for Anna as random, sourceless occurrences. We would have to point out, for years, that sound comes from people and things. And her brain would learn to "hear" very differently from a hearing person's; it would have to learn to *decode* electric impulses into intelligible, intoned sounds, with a lot of help from us, an auditory-verbal therapist, and an audiologist, who would program the devices to match Anna's brain and its changes every few months.

The audiologist asks if I have any questions, and I have so many, I say no. I want to talk to Luke and my mom. I want to begin being with Anna anew.

———

In the cold, covered parking lot, while Anita walks toward a rectangle of sun, I dial home.

"Mom." I try to steady myself but can't. My voice rises, tight, and I hear it, hear the sound of me that I'd always thought Anna had, too: "She's deaf."

On the other end of the line, I can sense the gaping fissure opened by our mutual grief and our inability to cover this cavity between us, to cry together, to embrace. There is nothing then, for a few seconds, but I know she's there. This silence is the pain of having to accept what's actual and true. "Oh, honey," she finally says, crying. "Have you told Luke?"

On the way back to the hotel, I ride in the back of the car with my phone, waiting to make the call. Part of me wants to be with Luke when I tell him. I want to be close enough to be held. But I also know he's waiting to hear how the appointment went. I'm watching Anna, and her eyes are following everything—the planes still spinning through the sky, the light igniting the bridges and the boats, the houses and trees and beauty that does not depend on sound. It is late afternoon by then, which means Luke will probably be in range, so I push his name on my screen.

"Hi!" he says, his optimism crushing me before I speak. I can hear the growl of his engine in the background, the plucky bluegrass of the satellite radio, and Luke asking me to wait just a minute while he cranks in a fish. How will Anna do all this? How will she use a phone? How will she span distance through language? How will she function in a hearing, talking, sound-filled world? When Luke returns, I tell him point-blank:

"Luke, she's deaf."

It's a simple thing to relay, without need for questions or answers. Deafness is hard to accept, not difficult to deliver.

"Wow," he says. Then it takes him some time to speak again. "I guess I just didn't think she'd be *deaf*-deaf, not all the way."

I can sense, in the silence that follows, a mixture of shock and sorrow, the first time since Anna's diagnosis that the gravity seems to be weighing on us with equal force.

"I know," I say. "I didn't, either."

The world is suspended, muted, watery. I have the sensation of floating as we drive. To say it feels surreal would be accurate, but it would also diminish the visceral way the news has scooped something out of my body, torn something painfully away, and yet created a new, explorable space. There's a buoyancy of relief here, as though some of CMV's secret has been exposed, concretized. No more clever tricks—Zaley yelling behind a closed door so Anna can't see her move, and us guessing if she heard. Anna can't hear, and that's it.

I ask myself how I'd not seen this coming—to the extent that I was *eating candy* when they delivered her diagnosis. I feel guilty for not using more signs, for not erring on the side of caution that Anna had always heard nothing, and I think of every hearing screener and audiologist who'd said *It's probably birth fluid* or *Don't worry, we'll try again,* and how misleading this is for those of us whose children are congenitally deaf. I'm saddened that our optimism meant a wrongful assumption about our daughter's innate qualities, as though we'd been protecting ourselves from her actuality instead of accepting it as an option, unconditionally, when she'd first surfaced silently out of me.

But there's something else here, too, a knifelike thought: a terror that if CMV could fully take away her hearing, maybe it's already taking away other abilities while we remain hopeful, resistant to every possibility, saying things like *Let's just wait till we have more information.*

My mom calls again, and when I answer, she asks what the ophthalmologist said. I had almost forgotten the interaction entirely: at the end of the audiology appointment, the providers had said their farewells, and I had, too, but I stayed sitting. They looked at each other nervously. "What about her eye appointment?" I'd asked. One audiologist leaned over the keyboard and clicked around, then shook her head. "I don't see an appointment here."

After a quick call, the eye doctor came down from another floor of the building and said she was sorry, she just couldn't fit us in. Then she stood in the doorway and, with a thick textbook in her hand, read to me the various ways blindness by infection could take the place of my daughter's sense of sight.

―――――

Back at the hotel room, Luke's dad, Willis, opens the door, expectant and hopeful, and I tell him that Anna is 100 percent deaf. He hugs me tight, then takes Anna from me and speaks to her like he always has. He lays her on the bed and smiles at her. He rolls her onto her tummy and remarks that she already looks stronger than she did a month ago—"Look, she's lifting her head!" She looks like a cartoon caterpillar with her Japanime eyes, her green gingham onesie, and her low-strength limbs.

When she makes the slightest sound of discontent, Willis carries Anna to the window where they stand for a long time, both quiet, looking at the boats skating across the white snakeskin surface of the lake.

"I think she's going to be just fine," he says, still looking out at the day.

He means it. It's heartbreaking and consoling. I believe him and I don't. He says what Luke would have said if he'd been able to come.

―――――

Later that night we have dinner at a fancy steak restaurant on the water with Luke's brother Gabe, who lives in Seattle. The fourth-youngest but biggest of all six boys, at six foot four Gabe is a smiling and gentle giant who dwarfs Anna as she sleeps against one of his biceps (which we'd once measured to find it was larger in circumference than my thigh). While we eat, floatplanes buzz down from the sky and land on the water that laps rhythmically against the deck of the restaurant. The sun goes down with more observable drama than we ever see in the midnight-sun of Sitka, turning Washington's sky into bursting apricot stripes. I finish a heavy, core-warming beer, and we walk the docks where yachts and wooden canoes yaw peacefully in pitch-black water.

But after we return to the hotel and everyone else is sleeping, a dark curiosity blows into me, ashlike, piling up in my limbs and my core. What if Anna is already going blind?

I imagine having to communicate with her, Helen Keller style, if she loses her ability to see. But then I realize: Helen Keller didn't have cognitive or fine motor delays, as Anna might, which could preclude her from even being able to sign.

I know that some mothers are burying their children with CMV, and that the privilege of language is just that. But my gratitude for Anna's life doesn't diminish my fears about her future. As a writer and reader, I find the prospect of a life void of language terrifyingly bereft. According to the memoirist Patricia Hampl, "A writer wishes—certainly we all wish—to speak about profound matters that are, like it or not, general and abstract. We wish to talk to each other about life and death, about love, despair, loss, and innocence. . . . We seek a means of exchange, a language which will renew these ancient concerns and make them wholly, pulsingly ours."

Yes. This is what I am prematurely mourning for Anna: the ability to identify the profound, to exchange depth with others, to renew, through language, the mundane. A life and concerns that are *wholly, pulsingly* hers.

But then I think of Bailey, the child with CMV in Alaska, and of what her mother had written: *She was social without communicating. She loved without words.*

Who was I to think that Bailey's life, Bailey's feelings, weren't wholly, pulsingly hers?

As I lie next to Anna, listening to the distant engines of cars driving through the Seattle night, I do feel that my love for her and hers for me is on a level higher, more transcendent than speech. I can feel this connection in the silence, as vital and wordless as the movement of our mutually infected blood.

All Anna's doctors have told us that she will likely be late to do everything and that we should prepare ourselves for the type of patience and altered timeline this requires. But they haven't said any-thing about the light speed of love—how it won't take any longer for us to love Anna or for Anna to love us.

I decide: if Anna has been such a source of profundity in my life, then she must contain the profound within her. And I have to believe that her experience of the world will be as deep as any, no matter her language, no matter that it might not have any outward shape, no matter that it might not look like mine.

———

People always play that game: would you rather be deaf or blind?

Deaf, deaf, deaf, I think then, knowing it's an unfair game, but feeling desperate for the function of Anna's eyes, which are half-open in the city-lit night. In desperation, we often revert to unrealistic wagers, and that night mine is: *I'll accept her deafness, God. But you have to let her see. I'll listen better. I'll stop gossiping. I'll be better at letting Luke be silent, too.*

"What's wrong?" I'll often say to Luke when he gets home tired, and I'm overly ready to talk.

"Nothing," he'll say.

"If nothing's wrong," I'll say, "then why aren't you saying anything?"

"I'm just *being* with you."

"Why do I always have to carry the conversation?"

"I always talk to you."

"Not as much as I talk to you."

Once I admitted, during confession, my tendency to force Luke into more talking—even if that meant fighting—and the priest said: "You're probably the one person who offers Luke the comfort of not having to talk."

He was right, and it stings me now to realize it: that I had often rejected the gift of silence; that silence did not mean less love.

The world, in fact, is already offering a soundless shelter for Anna. My priest brother, David, has enlisted thousands of people in what he's calling a "Thermonuclear Novena"—54 days' worth of special prayers for Anna shortly after her diagnosis with CMV. I've been trying to remember to pray it once a day. Most days I forget. Or

I get distracted by wondering if "ask and ye shall receive" is literal or what. Most of the time, mid-novena, I fall asleep.

Others are praying for Anna's total healing, and I love that they're thinking of her, that their appeal stems from care and concern. But already I can tell theirs is a different prayer than the one that's been forming tentatively inside me—a prayer of silence, a prayer *as* silence, that is many years out from my understanding. What I do know is, if I picture Anna as hearing, if I picture her without CMV, I'm not picturing a baby I know and love.

———

Part of me hates the thought of cochlear implants, the unnecessary severing of Anna's skin and the insertion of something inauthentic to her being. But I can't imagine what my life would be like without music. My memories contain a lifetime of it, and that night in Seattle, the songs engulf me, parade past me like people say their lives do during a near-death experience.

My grandma singing *Candy, I call my sugar candy;* the ragtime and '50s songs my dad plays on the organ. My mom's John Denver and Simon and Garfunkel LPs. My brother David playing the guitar, and my brother Michael playing the drums, and me watching from the basement staircase in middle school, jealous and proud. And the seven years I'd spent in New Orleans—going to college and then teaching—where music pumped through every moment like the city's heartbeat and blood.

Then there is Luke's voice alone, the first part of Luke I knew, his timbre somewhere between a bass and a tenor, his hold on a harmony a flow without detectable effort. There are the sounds of his music-making family, too: his mom belting out Earth, Wind & Fire while she cleans; the sound of her father, Papo, singing Frank Sinatra's "Sentimental Journey" at our wedding reception; Luke on the banjo, and any of his brothers on guitar, and all of them together like a modern family Von Trapp (minus girls).

I hear, in my head, the Neil Young songs we listen to on Luke's boat and at home in his truck. And Sharon Jones and Sade and John Prine—the voices I love when I'm alone that draw up moments from my past and fix them with more significance into who I am. Then I picture my childhood as a dancer, transcribing every type of music into movement, twisting and rising above a resin-coated floor, like a bird flying, like someone other than the bound person I was. And having moved like this, and borne girls, those are years and feelings I can't help but project into the lives of my daughters.

But Anna is deaf. Anna is *deaf*. Will she ever be lifted up, as I'd been, on the magnificent, weight-bearing wings of sound?

———

It's approaching morning in the crisp white bed. I haven't slept. Anita must hear the sound of my strained inhale, because she comes over to my side. She runs her hand up and down my back, as my mom used to do at night, when I was a child and wanted a few more minutes of company before I drifted off. There are no words, just the feeling of Anita's fingers, up and down, the extraction of pain through the recognition of it, and I know that if all I can give Anna is my touch, she will feel it, she will feel love, and for now, that has to be enough.

8

Flying back to Sitka, I watch the sun skip over the water, the frothy coasts, the white-rimmed islands. Luke is already out catching salmon while we fly over another country, bypass ancient glaciers, watch the boats below dividing the blue. How can the world go on turning, melting, working as usual, while my life is so irreparably altered?

The woman next to me has two girls in the seats behind us, and they are cooing to Anna, taking turns looking at her through the space between the seats. "She is really something," the woman says. "Look at that face of wonder!" It's the perfect expression for Anna—she is pure wonder, and maybe even more so because of the way she is.

"She's actually deaf," I tell the woman. "I just found out on this trip."

She looks straight at me, then back down at my baby. And instead of responding with pity, she places her palm on Anna's cheek, leans in close to her, and whispers, "Aren't you amazing?"

I'd expected Sitka to be surrounded by its usual force field of drizzle and fog. But as we approach town, we continue to be blessed by a bursting, well-defined sun. Inside the airport, I collect Anna's car seat from the conveyor belt and snap it back into our Suburban in the parking lot where you never have to pay to leave your car overnight. My keys are right where we always leave them in Sitka: in the ignition.

When I get to Jules's house, her kids and Zaley are, as promised, eating chocolate-studded pancakes at the kitchen table, as happy as ever. Luke has already told the news to Jules and her husband Derek, who heads Luke's four-boat fleet, and I can tell Jules is trying hard to hold back the tears. Zaley is ecstatic to see us, and she wants to know about Anna's ears.

"Anna is fine, sweetie," I tell Zaley. "But her ears don't work. She can't hear us."

"Even if we're loud?" Zaley asks, her voice getting louder as she says it.

"Even if you're as loud as you can be."

It seems like she understands at first. But a few minutes later, when Zaley is talking to Anna like always, "Hi baby, I missed you, I love you," and lifting Anna's arms up and down rapidly, I realize she won't understand for a long time that Anna is different.

Zaley's acceptance of Anna has been one of the greatest lessons of my motherhood. Not at the beginning and not ever after has Zaley rejected or questioned anything different about her sister. She has never wished that Anna could hear (in fact, Zaley has always wanted Anna's flashy devices for herself). She rejoices anytime Anna does something new and coaches her with unflagging energy, not believing there's any other option than for Anna to succeed.

Back at our house, while I unpack and fret from a distance about Anna, who is lying on the bed—*Will she ever roll over? Will she ever hold up her head?*—Zaley places props near Anna's body to encourage her to roll, dances dolls in front her and gives them silly voices, despite Anna's deafness. She exemplifies, in fact, the professional advice the audiologist had given me in Seattle: "Speak to Anna all the time. Speak to her as though she's hearing. A lot of parents find out their child is deaf, and they stop verbalizing to them. This is very much to the child's detriment."

Speaking to Anna as if she's hearing is the easiest thing ever. I only need to follow my instincts and Zaley's singsong, day-long monologues. Plus, speech is not just speech; it's a combination of facial expressions and gestures and mouth shapes, all of which Anna is still taking in, albeit without sound. Her eyes seem to widen and brighten by the day. She looks at me, and her lips turn up at the corners, almost conspiratorially. She is five weeks old. She is smiling already.

———

We can hear the FedEx man, spinning and grinding up the hill, before he delivers the packages, smiling, at our door. One of the boxes is from an herbalist in a Colorado mountain town: a tincture of lemon balm (a natural antiviral) and astralagus (an anti-inflammatory herb) for me to take twenty minutes prior to nursing. Via Amazon: a one-pound jar of phosphatidylcholine, a mitochondria-repairing powder that a naturopath recommended by phone and that I plop by heaping tablespoon into my smoothie every morning.

Anna's godmother, Natalia, sends clothes for both girls and coloring supplies and expensive face lotion (for me!), and she calls, offering a specific kind of empathy: her first daughter, now ten, was diagnosed as an infant with a rare and usually terminal kind of cancer called neuroblastoma. Alexis has been in remission for over nine years, but Natalia knows what I can already feel: that anxiety never goes into remission in a mother.

From Kodiak, my friend Sara—who now has two boys and a little girl—sends something funny or sustaining every month: googly-eyed slugs her boys molded from clay; colorful stationery; a poignant short story by Anne Carson about swimming.

My brother Michael and his wife, Brenda, send caring voicemails for me. They text silly pictures for Zaley of cats photoshopped and perched on top of family members' heads. My brother David mails us Padre Pio oil and passages from the Bible about suffering. My other friend Sarah, who has just been through a brutal divorce, emails me striking images of the Virgin Mary enduring a mother's most searing pain. Her face shows agony and ecstasy—the two emotions that coincide when we love as hard as we can.

I have always struggled to escape whatever immediate problem stands before me, and these images help. I do think of Mary in this line of other mothers who have struggled so gracefully as to make me feel alone in the sometimes ugly way I shoulder my sorrow. I remind myself that I am less important than all the suffering in the world that Anna's suffering has made me notice.

A friend needs a blood transfusion. A friend of a friend, a mother with young children, loses her hearing entirely and without warning.

An ecstatically expecting sister-in-law miscarries. A child with congenital CMV on the other side of the country dies at the age of five.

———

What I don't know, when I wake up on August 18, is that the water hammering down the creek outside and the water now howling down the windows is averaging four inches per hour. What I don't know when I text a friend who's out of town—*wow, you are missing quite the storm*—is that a few miles away, the mountain named Gavan has just fallen down.

Wide-eyed next to the window, Zaley and I eat eggs and toast. We watch the width of the rivulets change on the glass. A few hours later, when the rain changes to a trickle, the sun also appears, so we take advantage and go for a walk.

In our front yard, the little creek has become a powerful gushing thing the color and opaqueness of a Frappuccino. Purple fireweed petals are spinning down from Eliason Loop—the street perched on a shelf of stone above ours. The world is rinsed and reemerging in the sun. But what I don't know is that three people in our town are already gone.

In Sitka, there's no TV station that you can turn to when seeking the current weather or emergency reports. In the event of a landslide, you wait for news to landslide, too—by text, by phone, by neighbors who knock and then come inside for an hour. There's also a Facebook page called "Sitka Chatters," where people joke and hate and appreciate each other, and there's the website for the newspaper in town.

On our walk down the hill, a friend texts me a link to an article in the *Sitka Sentinel*: there's a picture of the familiar mountain, now fractured. There are already pictures of the missing—a middle-aged man I recognize, and two brothers in their twenties who go to the Catholic church. The police are issuing a mandatory evacuation of the area just under the slide. But on the other side of town, where we are right now standing on another compromised slope, there's no recommendation to find solid ground.

Zaley's asking why we we're stopped in the middle of the street, and while I want to run home and pack a bag and fly us off the island, I know I need to gather my wits against my instinct to run. I look up at the vertical magnitude of Mount Verstovia, imagining myself into its darkness and soil. Is the bedrock shifting now, and we don't know it? What unforeseeable event—wind, rain, another diagnosis—is going to bring me to my knees?

My phone beeps again. My friend Lisa Jean, a third-generation Sitkan whose mom taught me how to sew, has just taken her son to pull crab pots in Nakwasina Sound. She has taken pictures of the suture from her boat. I gasp at the images she's sent. The landslide is much larger than I'd pictured. Its darkness and width make me shudder—I'll find out later that the slide wiped out twelve acres—and I'm struck, as well, by its permanence: looking at that mountain, I realize its slope will never be the same.

The rain starts again. We turn around. A Coast Guard helicopter flies so low we can see the pilot's face. The sounds of those blades will continue for days as they search for signs of instability, and as scientists from NASA fly in to reassess where in Sitka people ought to live. At home, I watch the sky and listen to the radio where a reporter named Robert Woolsey says the landslide in Sitka is "a reminder that we live in this remarkable place at the mercy of forces beyond our control."

I think of this word *mercy*: to be "at the mercy" of something means we're defenseless, a victim in the shadow of much larger powers. But we are also deserving of mercy, of compassion, when we find ourselves in this position. This is the pattern of humanity: disaster followed by outpouring, loss met with love.

9

My friend Shelley invites us over. Also a mother and sometimes-writer, Shelley has two boys close in age to our girls. She works as a flight nurse, leaving the island a few times a month in an air ambulance, starting IVs at ten thousand feet and transporting people with medical complications off the island. Shelley and I met in the library when we were both first pregnant. Shelley was one of the few people who knew about CMV when I first told her Anna's diagnosis. She wanted me to write about it, and she wanted to read it.

Zaley and I slip off our boots on Shelley's side porch, which she has strung with bright fabric pennants. Inside, her house is humid and Shelley is pulling Dutch baby pancakes from the oven, puffy and golden in buttery glass pans.

"Sit down, friend," she says, pointing at the kitchen table, which is covered in Legos and crumbs. Shelley's house is never clean. But it's one of my favorite places in Sitka to be. There's a piano and a wood-burning stove and always the smell of something cooking. I sit down and take out my water bottle, cradling Anna in the nook of my left arm to nurse her. And that's when it happens.

I hear music. *Really* hear it. Like I am hearing it for the first time ever.

Ever since I returned from Seattle with my deaf child, I've intentionally withheld playing any music or going anywhere that it might be playing. Hearing it now is like being defibrillated at Shelley's table—a shock in the heart, a violent waking that I've been resisting every morning, afternoon, even while dreaming.

It's Emmylou Harris, and her voice is crooning from a speaker on the counter, so low and so layered with life and love and sorrow, it be that humans on both ends of the spectrum, though vulnerable and needy, are nearly transparent with mystery, contain some inexplicable proximity to what is unseen and true.

Back at the house, as I slip Zaley's watercolors and our photos from the fridge, I look at the pictures of me pregnant with Anna, and now I see what was unseen. I know CMV is like going upstream, partly broken, to experience something excruciating and glorious and life-bending that I will never fully understand.

We will leave behind this summer like we leave behind every summer: glad that fishing season is over but knowing that our girls will never be that young in Alaska again. It's time to do what Luke has taught me about accountability: no matter how many days you live somewhere or how tired you are, you get up early, you make the coffee. You talk to people with generosity even when you don't feel like talking. You engage fully with a place, no matter its temporality, no matter if you're leaving, no matter if it's raining.

So using a hot pink, hand-me-down Barbie fishing rod, Luke catches Zaley one last fish at the brackish mouth of the river. We say our annual goodbyes, talk of how hard it is to leave a place even if staying would be harder. That night online, after we've packed up all our stuff and we're facing home and Anna's looming unknowns, I find these words online from a mother whose son has congenital CMV. "Our kids won't live common lives," she has written. "They'll live extraordinary ones."

PART III

COMPANY

"Without friends, even the most agreeable of pursuits becomes tedious."

SAINT THOMAS AQUINAS

I

We descend into Denver through flashes of silent lightning. We pull up to our house at midnight, and I'm in love. The house is white, the door is red, the crickets are clicking out their songs in our overgrown grass.

Luke lugs Zaley from her car seat and brings her up the narrow staircase to bed. I slide Anna out of the car, too, and bring her to the porch, where her eyes find mine in the light. I sign to her "home"— all four fingertips touching the tip of the thumb—and I bounce them against my temple then my chin, to indicate where we sleep and eat. She looks at me wide-eyed, not knowing that coming home this year is more than I can sign or explain.

Our house sits just west of Denver, in a small town named Wheat Ridge, where a working farm up the street sells vegetables, cash only, and small Italian groceries display rows of fresh bread, peppered salami, and rolled-up cannoli. We bought one of the original hundred-year-old farmhouses in the area, a year before I became pregnant with Anna.

And by farmhouse, I don't mean some Joanna Gaines masterpiece—there are no shiplap walls, no modern fixtures, no open concept here. All our rooms are small and separate, and the staircase is dangerously not to code. You have to step down four inches into the kitchen, and most of our guests trip the first time they walk out of the kitchen and into the hall. Shortly after we moved in, Luke had to prop up the basement with a tool that looked like a tire jack because the main floor bathroom was sinking below the sink.

During the day, though, light pours into every space, and in the family room, a swing hangs from a beam like the one in *Winnie the Pooh,* with a flat board for the seat and rope that Luke spliced together, then sealed with a flame (and which we'll use for Anna's therapies in the years to come). I've painted every room in the house—some are salmon, some navy blue, others maroon—and the dining room is a deep, earthy green I concocted with cans of paint left in the crawl space where we once found a cat. There's also a child-size attic with angled wooden walls that I made into a reading nook for the girls. I love this house even though it cracks and creaks and leaks because, unlike everywhere we've lived in Alaska, it's ours.

But now it feels different. When I bring Anna inside, the door-frames look too narrow for a wheelchair, and above the front door is a doorbell, and on the counter is a speaker for streaming music from my phone. Upstairs there are more reminders: a lullaby CD I'd left on her dresser, a white noise machine still plugged into her wall.

Anna is three months old. Everyone on the flight, painfully, had wanted to know if she'd just been born. She has no head strength yet, just the strength of my hand behind her head. Looking out the window, I can see Luke filling the freezers in our garage with fish, and I envy him the ability to manage tasks without being destroyed, as I am, by the inexorable changes of our lives.

I am tired, older-feeling than I am. But I also feel like I was only half awake before having Anna. I am a different kind of mother now, more wounded, more resilient. Because of Anna, I am more than I have ever been.

———

Anna's hearing aids are the color I expected them to be. Zaley thinks they look perfectly fancy. I'm proud of them, but I resent them. I like them, and they sadden me. Looking at Anna in her new rosy devices, the gravity hits me as gravity does, unforeseeable and unprovoked. Now I will have to readjust these things all the time. Now my child is not just my child. She has to wear something that didn't come with her body, built in. The hearing aids are the first manufactured sign that she's different.

But the biggest problem is, ironically, the noise that they make.

Whenever the aids aren't airtight in Anna's ears, they emit a metallic squeal. And because even delayed babies move all the time, rubbing their heads on the sides of car seats, couches, shoulders, and chests, the hearing aids are always screeching, always demanding that I stop what I'm doing and readjust them on her head. This noise, after just a few days, seems to be taking a toll on my brain.

The hearing aids also give me the sense of being surveilled. The audiologist at Children's whom we meet, a kind and brown-bobbed woman named Kirsten, shows us on her computer screen that hearing aids and cochlear implants are outfitted with sophisticated sound-tracking technology that will report to her how many minutes of the day Anna has been wearing the devices—and what specifically she's been hearing.

At future appointments, when Kirsten plugs Anna's hearing aids into the computer, a pie chart will pop up, meting out the minutes Anna has spent listening to specific things: speech, music, even background noises like the radio or TV. These values call out how you've spent your days—kind of like an audio-only Nanny Cam: *We see that you spoke to your child for four hours today.* Or, *Looks like you used a screen for an average of four hours a day.*

When I pick Zaley up from school and turn on *Letter Factory* so I can get Anna down for a nap, I can picture the pie chart's values expanding in an unfavorable direction. When Anna won't sleep at night and I have her downstairs with Luke and me while we watch something stupid on TV, I feel like we're burning through adult screen time we could have used more freely, unsupervised by her ears.

(These analytics don't show up if your husband happens to drive off with the hearing aids on top of the car, and you have to order another $8,000 pair.)

When I tell my close friend Mia, who's a hairstylist and the queen of pragmatic style, that I'm struggling to keep it together, that the ever-shifting hearing aids are the straw upon this milking camel's back, she pulls a pair of women's mustard-colored tights out of her bag. (Only Mia would have a pair of mustard-colored tights in her bag.)

She cuts one leg off the tights. Then, with scissors, she cuts a line lengthwise so the fabric opens twice as wide. With this spandex strip, she circles Anna's head, pinning her hearing aids in place, and ties the tights at her crown in a bow. There's no more squealing from Anna's head, at least, and I realize the irony: in the midst of trying to bring Anna sound, I'm pursuing more silence for myself.

———

I had pictured that being home would heal me. But most days, as soon as I pour my coffee and the baby is crying and Zaley is late for school and I've forgotten it's our day to bring snacks for the class, I'm not sure how I'll make it through the hour. Even after Zaley's at school, I'm too weary to readjust Anna's headband when she's pulled it over her eyes for the twentieth time, too defeated to rehang the heavy processors on the bendy rims of her ears. (CMV, ridiculously, can cause a lack of cartilage right there.) I feel hot and teary and so very alone.

I have Luke, of course, who collects stray sticks in the yard with Anna happily draped over his muscular left shoulder. But when I sit on the porch, on hold with whatever specialist we need to see next, I envy how easy fatherhood looks on him, and I wonder where I can find a similarly stressed, stay-at-home, CMV mom like me. Maybe she could bring her slightly older child who happens to be deaf. Maybe she drinks wine. Sometimes a little before five.

Multiple providers have promised they'll introduce me to another CMV family, but no one has. Not our early interventionist, who says she knows a number of other children with Anna's disease. Not Shannon Hughes, the PA at Children's who tells me at an otherwise uneventful appointment at Children's that Kristen Spytek, the mom who started the National CMV Foundation and who lost her daughter, Evelyn, to complications of CMV, lives in Denver—but because her husband is a scout for the NFL, their family is moving to Florida *this week*. And not our OT, who shows up at our front door, and whose face I immediately recognize: she's the operatic soprano in the Roman Catholic choir at St. Elizabeth's, where our Eastern church is housed.

I will end up loving all these providers, and I do believe they want to connect me. But they all offhandedly mention a problem with the system and their powerlessness against it: that problem is HIPAA—the Health Insurance Portability and Accountability Act, which sets boundaries on the use and release of medical records and ostensibly gives patients more control over their own information. But I don't feel like there's any centralization of Anna's information among all the specialists we've seen, and I'm starting to feel like HIPAA is, more than anything, securing my sense of isolation.

Gone are the days when a doctor or a therapist could say, "Here, let me give you this other mother's phone number." Now any provider needs permission before they provide that connection, even though meeting another CMV family would be more powerful right now, more healing for me, than a prescription. It seems we have created a medical system that protects our names and addresses at the cost of human connection.

I know that the Children's Hospital CMV Clinic has seen at least forty other families, this year alone. Which means there are hundreds, maybe even thousands of us in town with a diagnosis (not to mention the other 75 percent of children with congenital CMV in Colorado who are unidentified and undiagnosed).

And yet even those of us who know who we are remain siloed from each other—that extra email we've asked of a provider too much to remember alongside their mountains of obligatory paperwork.

When I look up the financial cost of HIPAA, I find numbers that confirm my suspicions: HIPAA was supposed to cost $14.5 million annually, but it actually costs closer to $8.3 billion a year. I read that individual doctors pay $35,000 a year to keep their technology compliant. And eventually I find an article, written by a physician named Kim Lien-Nguyen in *Medical Economics*, that explains the repercussions of HIPAA's astronomical costs: "HIPAA has impeded communication about risks to the public, contributed to inefficient care of patients by limiting physician communication, deterred medical research through the high costs of compliance, and stolen physician time from patients."

We are, essentially, paying our doctors not to discuss things like CMV, to conduct fewer studies, to limit the lengths of their consultations. I am alone, in large part, because we pay the medical system to cultivate silence.

I have loved Anna more each day of her life. I love her in absolutes that are not time or ability-dependent, that have nothing to do with past or future or present. The fact that she *is,* that she survived an invasion by a biological enemy that could have stopped her every everything, does not cease to rush through me as a plunging, submerging sort of revelation. I stand before her in the humility and amazement that accompany any goosebump-giving, life-transforming love story. But that doesn't mean I don't also notice how different she is.

Every morning when I bring Zaley to school, Anna is wearing her hearing aids, so I have to explain to the teachers and other parents—or whoever happens to compliment her signature headbands—that Anna is profoundly deaf. This generates a great, silent awkwardness.

Can she hear with the hearing aids, then? other mothers ask, hopeful, eager to hear that her problems have been solved. Then: *Oh . . . but she still needs to wear them?* Which is exactly the same question I ask myself every morning.

People also keep taking stabs at her age, followed by *Wow she's so small.* Or *Aw, she must be tired.* This is a remark Anna will get for years because one of her eyes doesn't open quite as wide as the other, and because sometimes you can see in her unblinking, fixed eyes just how hard she focuses, all day, on the shapes of other people's mouths to decipher what they're saying.

I want to tell these commenting mothers, *No, you look tired,* but I stop myself before I widen the gap between us that already exists. A child with visible needs can draw a pretty clear line between those who possess self-restraint and those who don't. Plus, I know most other parents are kind at heart, and I'd always rather talk about Anna than have people look at her, then look away. Anna's differences are both a bridge and a divide.

I do make a point to tell the parents of Zaley's peers that Anna was born deaf due to a common but dangerous virus I caught while pregnant called CMV. They probably think I'm a little intense, as I cover the million-year history of the virus in the time it takes to zip Zaley's coat. But all of them listen. They're appalled that they've never heard of CMV. And they want to know. Especially the preg-

answers that question I had in the beginning: *how does no one know?*

There's another child whose story is riveting to me, maybe because he's from Colorado, or maybe because his entry is so detailed, but I'm reading it quickly, skimming for information on how he's doing, until something is pulling up my eyes, and then I see—as my hand goes instinctually to my lips, as though this will prevent me from fully taking it in—that also listed, under his birthdate, is his deceased date. He died when he was three and a half years old.

His name is Jayden.

———

A week later, out of the blue, I receive a phone call from a number I don't know. It begins with a Colorado area code, so I answer.

It's Jayden's mom.

Her name is Karina. She'd seen my entry on the CMV registry. She's calling to invite me over, to meet Anna, to hand over any resources we might be able to use.

I say yes. Then I worry about it for days. Will this divide be too great between her severely ill, now-deceased child and my more moderately affected, still-living girl? I speculate about her motivations aloud to Luke: Does she actually want to meet Anna—an introduction I'm not sure I could, in her position, attempt? What kind of resources does she have that might be valuable to Anna's trajectory, and will these further overwhelm me? Or is she inviting me over because she feels she can reencounter a piece of Jayden in other children with CMV, similar to my desire to meet another baby with the same seemingly nonexistent disease? Maybe her invitation stems from the same longing I have for someone who just "gets it"—who gets the acronym without explanation, who gets the anxiety, who gets the rage, even if the feelings occurred for Karina in life-threatening circumstances, many years past. And can you even call that yearning for connection "similar," given the drastic differences of our experiences? I worry that Anna's aliveness might magnify the immensity of Karina's loss.

"Holy moly, just go over there, love," Luke says. "You'll be glad you did."

———

Snow is coating the roads, but Karina lives only ten minutes away. When I pull up to their house, her three young children are peering out the glass front door. They are four, three, and two years old. (Karina's now-oldest was three months old when Jayden passed away.) With one hand, Karina holds open the door, and one of the girls says her name is Zaley, and I'm speechless for a second, never having met another child with my daughter's name. It turns out she spells it differently—ZaiLie. But still.

Karina is younger than I'd expected—younger than me—with a face both hesitant and welcoming, tight curls, and glowing freckled skin. She's also Black, which is more relevant to the CMV experience than I realize at the time: per 1,000 live births, 3 white infants are infected with CMV versus 9.5 black infants. And Black children are up to twice as likely to die from CMV-related complications than white children.

This may be because Black women have less access to quality healthcare—which likely means most have less information about CMV or avoiding infection, in general, during pregnancy. But it is also true that even when well educated, Black women have worse birth outcomes in general than white women who haven't graduated from high school.

I want to hug Karina in her doorway, but she holds out her hand—not out of stiffness, I can tell, but out of shyness. Her kids take Zaley's hands, too, and lead her into their family room, where there's a wall-length bookshelf and photo albums lined up like rows of tall, uneven teeth. I can see, on most, the letters of Jayden's name.

Neither Karina nor I know how to begin. I sit on the floor and strip Anna's fleece polar bear suit from her rigid limbs. She's been doing this thing where she stretches her legs out and presses the soles of her feet together, like she's gripping a stick between her soles. I sit her up as much as I can between my legs and readjust her magenta headband.

"They told us to get cochlear implants for Jayden, but we never did," Karina says, knowing that Anna's hearing aids are likely a step in that direction. Then she says, "Gosh, she looks really good. She looks like she's doing really well."

"She is," I tell Karina. "We're really lucky."

But as soon as I say it, I disagree with it. *Lucky* has never felt like the right word to describe our experience. I certainly don't believe it's luck that proffered Anna to us without hip dysplasia or seizures, any more than I think it's bad luck that someone like Karina had a son as affected as Jayden and lost him.

When I turn my head to look for Zaley, I notice crosses hanging on many of the walls, and I feel their weight and significance. To know that Karina believes in something other than us as the generator of this complicated system of life, that she believes our children are more than mere entropic bundles of DNA, is to assume that she might think the same thing as me: that our children are born a specific way not by chance but because they are part of a more complete, incomprehensible picture, just as they are.

Do Karina and I both hate the cross that CMV is and wish it didn't exist, and do we both see a coming era in which it will never saddle any children with its side effects? Absolutely—and we've already expressed as much in our brief exchange. But our children are our children, and to say we love them is to say we love everything that makes them *them*: their deafness, their blindness, their pacing, their faces. In a complicated way, it may be true to say we love them because of CMV, not in spite of it.

This still leaves room for loathing the pain CMV puts our children through—the hospitalizations, the surgeries, the pain of their many recoveries. But the word *paradox* comes from the Latin word *paradoxum*, which means "seemingly absurd, but actually true," and it does feel both absurd and true that I wish CMV didn't exist, and yet I love what it's brought into my life: not just my daughter but this woman sitting on the floor, sharing her home with me, and asking to hold my child.

Karina takes Anna from me, unafraid of her fragility, and turns to face the albums on the wall. Then, with my daughter in one hand and the memories of her son in the other, she takes down every single album of Jayden to tell me about their life before him, and during, and after.

Karina was eighteen, newly married to her high school sweetheart, LeDaniel, when she got pregnant with Jayden. She expected what a lot of us expect: a baby who'd eat, smile, breathe, and sleep. Karina's dreams of typicality pivoted, though, before she even gave birth. She went into preterm labor at thirty-four weeks and was sent to a high-risk OB, where, hours before delivery, she found out that the baby growing inside her had incurred severe damage to his brain.

Later that day, in January 2008, Jayden was born weighing only three pounds. He was also born silent, like Anna and many other newborns with congenital CMV. He was immediately taken to the neonatal intensive care unit (NICU), where he underwent multiple tests and received a rare, prompt diagnosis of congenital CMV. But in the month he spent in the NICU, Jayden was never treated with antivirals—his parents wouldn't find out the medication existed until many years later.

He underwent blood transfusions and light therapy for extreme bilirubin, and he failed his hearing and vision screenings. "Not fully Helen Keller," Karina had written online when he was alive, "but he's almost fully deaf, and he is cortically blind, meaning he only sees light."

I'd read the longer version of Jayden's story on the National CMV Foundation's website before going to Karina's house. I was impressed by the narrative she'd written in real time: it was precise and hopeful, unembellished but profound. She'd written it in the moment, without reflection, adding onto it when he had major successes or setbacks, and it gave Jayden's life a jarring, present-tense nature—fitting for the moment-by-moment way Karina experienced the life and death of her son, and fitting for the way people should think about the disease, since every half-hour in the United States, a child is born with congenital CMV.

Jayden remained silent for almost a year, during which time his parents believed he was mute. During his massive seizures, which were picked up by EEG on day one but became outwardly detectable only at seven months, Karina wrote: "We are helpless as we hold him, trying to get him to breathe. He turns red and blue and goes limp," and here, anytime I revisit her words, my breath goes thin: "He wants help, but we can't give it."

———

For most of his childhood, Jayden had fifty to one hundred seizures a day. His doctors told Karina: "Every seizure, no matter if it's one minute or one hour, is taking time off his life." I picture being Karina when the doctors said this to her. I'm sure I would have felt that each of my child's seizures was taking time off my life, too. When Jayden was ten months old, he was placed on hospice. When he was two, his parents had to preplan his funeral.

And yet despite all his suffering, he lived—and he lived with volume and humor.

"He was nonverbal but very vocal," Karina remembers. "After his year of silence, he became so loud! He smiled all the time. He loved to laugh out loud at unexpected noises, and we'd make them for him just to see him light up and turn his head."

By the time Jayden was three, he was on fifteen daily medications. He had a vagus nerve stimulation pacemaker that sent continuous electric shock to his brain. He suffered from two dislocated hips (dislocating joints is common to low-toned children with CMV), an injured arm, and unpredictable blood sugar that could spike, then dangerously plummet.

Jayden never went to school. He never spoke a word. He wore overalls and loved the feel of the hammock, the latticed embrace of interwoven cords.

———

"I read some of Jayden's story, but I only saw one picture of him online," I admit to Karina while stopping on certain pages of her photo albums. I'm struck by his serene face in profile, by the scene of LeDaniel holding him way up high—Jayden in denim overalls and a Mohawk—against a dark blue Colorado sky.

Jayden was an objectively gorgeous child, with mature eyebrows, dark lips, and copper skin. His hair held tight curls like Karina's. In many of his pictures, Jayden looked happy, really happy—like he was laughing. There are pictures of him in the hospital, in parks, at home, at relatives' homes. "I love seeing these pictures of him in so many places."

I don't just love the images; I love how many there are. I love how much his parents captured both his suffering and his joy. Even though Jayden would never have ordinary cake-eating birthdays or be able to press a doorbell while trick-or-treating, he's surrounded in each picture by the happy trimmings of typical holidays. Pictures with lavish fondant on all his birthday cakes (though he'd never eat them, he could see the colors and candles on them); pictures with costumery and candy and decorations on Christmas and Easter and Halloween.

"We took him everywhere and did everything with him whether or not he could fully participate," Karina says, which seems strikingly compassionate, especially since I know some of the things they did with Jayden and all his equipment must have taken incredible energy. "The point," she says, "was to build an experience and memory."

Where some mothers might have kept a single album of their child who'd died young, before me is an anthology of what seems like every one of his days. And these aren't just photo albums; they're artistic collages, assembled with pinking shears and printed quotes, colorful frames and careful calligraphy, and no one book is less impressive than the others. Her devotion to Jayden is so holdable, so readable, I know that the collection in my lap is much more than just photographs; it's his whole life for her to share when she doesn't have her son to share anymore.

This is the answer, I now know, aching in the face of its obvious, beautiful simplicity: Jayden is the reason she invited me over.

———

Jayden looks nothing like Anna in his pictures, and yet looking at him is like looking at her. He has that far-off look: the distinction of illness or intelligence or some kind of discernment. His eyes are slightly atypical. They are outward-angled or even outward-seeking. Maybe it's me projecting the same qualities into him I've witnessed in Anna, but that doesn't mean what I see isn't true. Later, other mothers I find online will ask this same question: *Do you think our CMV babies look kind of similar? I can't put my finger on it, but some of your babies look like mine.*

Anna has always looked just enough different that people some-times comment, calling her exotic, or saying she doesn't look at all like our other children. Her face is small and ethereal and dusted with freckles. Her body is lighter than those half her age. Sometimes Zaley stares at Anna and says, "What is it about her? She's just so . . . beautiful."

As Karina remembers Jayden, her voice lopes without catching. But as I think of the first months of Anna's life, my throat lumps up. I'm not sure if I'm crying about Jayden's early death or if I'm crying about Karina's love or if I'm crying in shameful relief that Anna's eyes are still here for me to behold, that her back still radiates warmth against my abdomen, and that despite this virus, the synapses inside her are efficiently firing the dance of the everyday that we often fail to notice: eyelids blinking, hands closing and opening, the poetry of breath, pushing into me then pulling away.

———

According to Karina, Jayden's daily routine was: yell, smile, seize, OT. And always, always he loved to be held.

"Did I ever ask, *why me?*" Karina asks, then answers: "No. But I always asked, *why Jayden?* Why does he suffer so much each day? Why are these poor children born to die? We are all born to die, but I would much rather an adult who has lived their life go before these innocent children. No parent should have to go through this for their child.

"But I believe," she insists, "we were given him for a reason."

3

In a little-known, insightful document written in 1957 called *The Pedagogy of Innocent Suffering,* an Italian priest named Father Carlos Gnocchi attempted to answer the question of what we're to do with the unfathomable suffering of the innocent and the young. Gnocchi had seen his share of above-average tragedies, caring for starving and terribly wounded children in the aftermath of World War II. As many are tempted to do, including me, he could have renounced a God who could allow for such unfair cruelty in the world. But he saw suffering as exactly the opposite: he believed that to intimately experience and tend lovingly to suffering was a way to heal the brokenness of the systems and people from whom those atrocities originated.

To understand Gnocchi's perspective, you have to know how deeply he believed in the dignity—even the divinity—embodied by small children, especially those who had challenges or had been harmed. He cared for young boys who'd had their limbs and eyes blown out by landmines. He witnessed orphans in Yugoslavia banging dented plates, holding out tomato cans and boxes for food in the streets. He voluntarily enlisted in the war so he could comfort and continue to educate his young pupils before they were sent to Russia, where frozen white valleys would be plastered with the bodies of the dead. In these children and young men, he often witnessed a supernatural collision between the physical world and the spiritual—children seeing their own guardian angels or being acutely aware of a direct connection with God. In these children, he suggested, we can encounter something much more meaningful and vast than our singular, human experience.

"If suffering, according to the Gospel, reveals the presence of Christ in a man," he writes, "in no one is this made more transparent, clear, evident and immediate, than in the child." He then specifies: "To a child who suffers from a disability, deficiency, mutilation, poverty, sickness, ignorance, abandonment, or from any other cause, our internal disposition or external attitude should be dominated by a profound feeling of respect and veneration. I would almost say that it should be of worship."

This is a radical idea, even today: that the disabled are not just worthy of being included in politically correct advertisements, but perhaps they're of even more value to humanity than the children we consider typical or high-achieving. Maybe this is what Karina meant when she said they were given Jayden for a reason; he carved a fathomless depth in their loving, required not just vigilance but a profound, demanding way of living.

Gnocchi in no way detracted from the grave pain caused by suffering and bearing witness to suffering. In fact, he believed that all too often, bystanders of the bereaved try to placate those who suffer by calming them, distracting them, or diluting their pain. Rather than discounting sorrow, he writes that we have a deep obligation to unite the anguish of innocents to a more universal, love-driven cause—such as healing the social body—or else we are wasting a powerful opportunity for suffering children to feel that their lives are of inestimable import to the world.

In teaching others how best to serve children experiencing extreme strife, he wrote: "The pedagogy of suffering must, above all, teach children in a practical way to not keep their pain for themselves. But rather to give their pain as a gift to others." He suggests to direct "the pain or renunciation to concrete objectives, such as the healing of a loved one, to obtain an important grace, for the end of war," believing that "if there is a noble interest behind every pain of life, living will become both sacrificial and poetic."

Of course, Gnocchi's pedagogy is based on Christian teachings and the existence of Christ as the paradigm of meaningful suffering. But his insights seem convincing whether or not you're religious: that a suffering child's life would be less painful and moreover, even poetic, heroic, if they knew that their illness—that *they*—were of great significance.

Gnocchi says Saint Leonidas exemplified this veneration of children. Leonidas used to kiss the heart of his small child every morning, knowing this is where God was most present and at work. Reading this, I love my children even more. And I want to be a parent like him.

———

No matter how much suffering a child appears to have gone through, of course, no one can really measure the quantity, the poundage of their trials. That's why some mothers of medically complex children make "warrior beads" for them: a necklace with beads that denote each hospital visit, stay, or surgery. Some of these necklaces are hundreds of beads long. Jayden's would have been heavy, colorful, replete.

Throughout his short life, CMV was lying dormant in the cells of his body, always waiting for the opportunity to reactivate. Like the herpes virus that causes cold sores, once someone has their first CMV infection, the virus then goes quiet in their system, reactivating during times of stress over the course of their lifetime. Most healthy people wouldn't even be aware they were experiencing a CMV reactivation, but for children like Jayden, who have more fragile immune systems, a reactivation can be devastating. The sicker Jayden became, the more CMV ran rampant in his system, attacking his organs and decreasing his lifelong capacity to fight illness. He had a two-hour seizure and was tended to by five doctors and six nurses before an adult critical care doctor placed a central line in his groin that finally stopped the seizure. After that, Jayden endured a month-long hospital stay and a handful of surgeries, including the introduction of a G-tube because he never regained the ability to eat. The stories of so many children with CMV go like this: one thing after another, a slow slide toward slowing down forever.

Right after his third birthday, Jayden started to reject G-tube feedings, too, and consequently, his stomach and digestive systems entered an early phase of shutting down. After ten days without food, his lungs filled with fluid, and he took a breath only every forty-five to sixty seconds. Then his kidneys shut down, and finally, his circulatory system failed to move. On August 13, 2011, after twenty-four days without eating—a feat that amazed his doctors—he refused his oral pain meds. Karina remembers the day as unbearably long. By eight p.m., he was not clearing the fluid that had been bubbling around his mouth. Karina took him and held him. She knew he was drowning.

"He looked terrified," she wrote. "We held him close and told him it was okay to go. We looked down at one point and saw his baby brother holding his arm."

Six minutes later Jayden's heart stopped. Karina closed his eyes. She sat still. She held him. Her first son, his body released from the trouble of living.

While she waited for the hospice nurses to arrive, Karina tidied Jayden, slipped him into his favorite pajamas—baseball-themed and lightweight on his tube-punctured abdomen, with white and navy blue stripes. When two kind men from the mortuary showed up, they opened the doors to their van, and Karina saw with an unexpected burst of comfort that they'd made up a bed in the back with teddy bears and soft blankets just for Jayden. Karina's husband carried Jayden out.

And then they said goodbye to their baby.

"Not many adults could have dealt with the things our three-year-old could and did," Karina wrote, after his death. "He is at peace now. He is whole and healthy. He is our angel. We miss him dearly."

———

There's one particular passage in *The Pedagogy of Innocent Suffering* that strikes me most in relationship to Jayden and CMV: it's a parable about a little bird who could bear the load of disease and eventually heal the sick.

In this parable, a person who was suffering greatly from the effects of jaundice lay down to grieve in the shade of a tree. Up in the boughs, an unassuming bird kept vigil over the ill. This bird, though small, began to take on the sick man's yellowing hue. And as the bird absorbed the jaundiced man's pain, the sickly color drained from the body suffering under the tree. Finally, when the bird had become a raging yellow and the sick man had been completely restored to his natural color, the little bird sang a song of farewell and retreated in its full plumes of color, to die.

I wonder if it's possible that children like Jayden, who have an abundance of CMV symptoms, are drenched in color for the world to see. They carry the visibility of the disease for those of us who don't. Without them, without their deep affliction, we would never *see* congenital CMV. And we would not have any progress, slow though it may be, toward healing CMV—including naming it, treating it, and preventing the next generation from contracting it.

As C. S. Lewis writes, pain is God's "megaphone to rouse a deaf world."

———

Years later, when I press Karina, who's now an ICU nurse, about what she meant when she said Jayden was given to her for a reason, she says, "There's just a feeling of peace and closeness when I'm caring for patients who walk the thin line between life and death. Jayden made me separate the important things from the unnecessary things in life. I feel called to do more for others as a way to honor him. I feel compelled to seek God."

———

When I leave Karina's house, the snow is falling plentifully, in visible hexagons that seem to spin down in slow motion, as if in a dream. My girls are tired and quiet and we drive home over hilly, wet streets where the snowflakes disappear as soon as they touch the road. I can't bear the idea of going home, being inside, awaiting the banality that will inevitably overtake this state of awareness, this proximity to death and to life. I want to be washed in the wordlessness and place-warp of however much snow is going to fall.

So we drive and drive around the side of the city that Karina and I share, and I think of her warm home and how hard she loves her children, and I think of Jayden in my favorite picture as he lay in that hammock, his eyes closed, his lips slightly upturned and content, and I wonder what he saw when he saw light. I wonder if inside his eyes, it was like a heavy snow.

Anna stays asleep longer on this drive than she has in the car since

think of sounds in a visual sense, in colors, she writes.

———

It's a loud day when I end up calling Lee. I'm sitting on my parents' porch, Anna is asleep in the back of my car with the windows down, and across the street, a company is sawing and grinding the branches of a cottonwood tree. I ask Lee to tell me the story of her Anna, of her experience with CMV.

"I just remember in the beginning, I was so angry," she says. "I was so mad that no one had told me about CMV."

I can tell that Lee means she's still angry, and she explains: she isn't just upset about her Anna, she's upset about mine—that two decades later, with the swift dissemination of information through the internet and major advancements in infectious disease, I've still given birth to a baby with CMV without any knowledge it exists.

"I've always been more upset about CMV than my daughter has, which is a blessing," Lee says. "Actually, Anna has never been impeded by her deafness. Really, her motor delays have been more prohibiting than being deaf ever has. She loved swimming, riding horses, and playing piano and golf, but because one side doesn't work as well as the other—a symptom called *hemiparesis*—she eventually had to give in and accept that she can't do them well. These limitations set her apart from her peers far more than her being profoundly deaf."

This chips a little notch in my heart. Moderate gross motor delays are a different kind of struggle, of course, than the child who undergoes ten years of therapy to eat solid food or sit up. But watching your child alter course due to any inability will heavy the heart, whether they're a toddler or a teen, disabled or not.

Lee's daughter Anna looks like any college-age girl. She's the type of sunny person with big spiraled hair and a big genuine smile whom you might see and think, *Man, life must be so easy for her.* But Anna's challenges are the kind you can't see: she's had to battle the tease of a seemingly typical body that isn't actually typical when it applies itself to the things she wants to do. And I happen to love swimming and horses, too.

———

I spent all day, every day of my childhood summers swimming, both for fun and on the neighborhood swim team. But once I was in high school and too old to enjoy the water all day for free, my next-door neighbor, Karen, and I found work at a nearby club where the members boarded and rode forty-some horses. Every day we'd meet on the sidewalk in the gold-gray of dawn and drive ten minutes together to a more affluent neighborhood, where we'd spend the day shoveling shit and bringing out to pasture horses that other people owned.

Neither of us came from families where we could have afforded a riding hobby—or even dreamed of one—but we were granted the thrill of exercising the horses at the club if their owners were injured or had no interest in caring for their charge. Karen rode a horse whose owner had broken her back. The horse I rode, named Heidi, was a castoff from the agricultural program at Colorado State University; she would end up pregnant, giving birth at midnight to a glistening foal, the most fragile life I'd yet beheld.

As a bonus for our hard work, a riding instructor agreed to give us lessons for free after we were finished with Saturday morning feeds. So we learned to ride English and then bareback, and after our lessons, we took our mares on a gravel path along a slow brown canal to a meadow that opened, shimmering and flaxen, before us. That's where we ran wild—cantering and galloping and stopping for our breath, more ourselves, more full than we'd been anywhere else. Then we'd walk back, talking and patting the horses' necks, before untacking, curry-combing their sweat-stained backs, and feeding them all again.

———

Riding was more than fun. It was a way of feeling power at a time in my life when my personal worth felt compromised by the clothes, bodies, and abilities of others. Karen's body was more developed, better shaped than mine. I knew this when we went to the pool, when we tried on each other's clothes, when the boy I loved liked her instead of me. But on the horses, I could ride away from Karen's body, away from my jealousy, away from everything. Horses demand that your attention barely leaves yourself or your horse. Those horses taught me balance and self-respect, and they healed something in me I couldn't quite name.

Watching Anna's chest rise and fall under her car seat straps, I know her limbs might be different, less obedient, thinner than mine. I just want her opportunities to be as numberless as the reeds in those horse-trodden fields.

"Had you ever heard of congenital CMV?" Lee asks me.

"No. I didn't even know the definition of the word *congenital* till she was diagnosed."

And now I know it doesn't just mean "from birth"; it means CMV will impact our children until their deaths.

Then Lee tells me a story to lighten the tone. On Anna's first day of college, she didn't realize it, but she didn't have fully charged batteries in her cochlear implants. By midafternoon, she had to explain to her professors and peers—who had no idea she was deaf—that she needed to excuse herself because she couldn't hear a thing. But Anna had laughed it off and started calling the internal warning sound that cochlear implants emit right before they die "the beep of doom."

I have one more question for Lee—something that is gnawing at me, just the slightest bit, because I want to talk to Luke about it. "After you had Anna," I ask her, "did you have other kids?"

"We had Anna before doctors know what they know now," Lee says, and only now do I hear full-blown sorrow over the phone. "While we felt strangely fortunate that Anna's CMV caused only deafness and hemiparesis, back then, our doctors had never seen a known case of CMV. So all we knew was the textbook rendition of debilitating and, in many cases, life-threatening conditions the virus could cause. We were so terrified we'd have another child with CMV, we never did."

───────

And so I alternate between the experiences of the living and the memories of the deceased. Between the intellectually disabled and those earning degrees. Between the hearing world, where we live, and that of the Deaf community (in which the capital *D* means people who use sign language and identify culturally as being Deaf), which I have yet to experience or even see.

Until, back at our house, the doorbell rings.

Lori is in her fifties. Her thick hair is both blond and brown, and it shakes at her shoulders when, in the threshold of our front door, she signs *hello*—a straight hand coming off the forehead, almost like a military salute. Lori's services have been provided to us for free, by the state, through a program at the Colorado School for the Deaf and the Blind, where a Deaf mentor will teach us sign language once a week, in our home, till Anna turns five.

Lori hugs me tight right away, in the doorway, as if we already know and like each other. When I step back to let her in, she walks into our kitchen, looks around the corner at the family room, and around the other corner to the dark green dining room, and signs *beautiful*—a hand encircling the face—a sign I only know from watching *Mr. Holland's Opus* twenty-some years ago.

I actually know a few other signs, and not just from the YouTube videos and *Signing Times* episodes I've been watching since July. At my Catholic grade school, we'd learned to recite most of our prayers in American Sign Language, or ASL, sitting in an attentive circle on the floor. I remember the entirety of the "Our Father," our teacher explaining the logical representations of words like *forgive*—a hand wiping the other as clean as a slate; *trespass*—two index fingers pushing against each other, the same sign as for *injury;* and *kingdom*—a *K* slung from shoulder to opposite hip, like a hand-width royal sash.

Sign language seemed immediately warm and welcoming, more accessible than any foreign language I could learn. And in many ways, it is—a foreign tongue feels more daunting than an open hand. I loved how my teacher's fingers made a shape I'd never thought to make, how I could hold that word by making it myself. I loved the way my hands became faster as I practiced, as if language were an athletic endeavor. I loved that my brothers hadn't learned sign language since they had a different religion teacher, so ASL was mine and mine alone.

At home, based on the all the words in the prayers I knew, I'd put sentences together as a linguistic game while lying in bed at night. *Lead me, fruit. On earth, we eat bread. Heaven has a name.* I remember a feeling of limitation followed by yearning—a hopefulness that one day I might be fluent.

———

If you're hearing, it's hard not to speak when you try to communicate initially with someone who's Deaf. So I gesture to Lori awkwardly, like I'm some English butler, directing her to the family room where there's a leather couch and two upholstered chairs, and I say, quietly, knowing I'm not being heard, "We can sit in here."

But Lori doesn't seem awkward at all. Instead of sitting on the furniture, she sits right down on the rug—where she's used to working with children—and takes some papers out of her purse. When I sit down on the ground with Anna, Lori has no hesitation. Her hands are already flowing, articulating, showing my daughter a path to self-expression.

Language acquisition is mysterious, gradual, leaving no hard, fast memory of how it sticks to the brain. How do Lori and I, Lori and Luke, Lori and our children understand each other without a shared glossary? How does her knowledge locate our readiness? How is her gift so seamlessly imparted? I'm not exactly sure. Sometimes she brings flash cards, points to a picture, then signs it in the air. Sometimes she points at objects around the house, or colors on our clothes. Sometimes we finger-spell when we can't translate each other's expressions. Lori is a lively, nonjudgmental, open window into the life of my exceptional child.

When I ask her questions about motherhood as a Deaf woman, she explains how she woke to her boys when they cried in the night as infants. (A vibrating pad underneath her mattress shook the bed when the baby monitor made a sound.) When her doorbell rings, it lights up a bright flashing light. She explains that even though her children are hearing and speaking, their first language was ASL. She tells me about coffee shops nearby where the baristas know some Sign, dentists for the Deaf, and vets who use ASL. Sometimes we chat smoothly for over an hour, nodding our hands and lifting our eyebrows, friendship the language that traverses our differences.

Over the weeks, vocabulary accumulates. Like grade school units about the pyramids in Egypt or the solar system or the seder meal, entering into another world is a feasting: *possum, snail, hippo, chicken.*

Island, mountain, cloud, and *ocean. Embarrassed, happy, brave, excited. Luke is silly. Zaley is jumping. Anna is watching.*
    I am Mom. You're my girl. I see you. I hold you. I love you.

———

Two Fridays a month, the Rocky Mountain Deaf School, known as RMDS, holds a toddler program for children who are deaf or hard of hearing, and Lori has suggested we attend. Luke is hunting during the first week of the program, so I ask my mom if she'll come with me and the girls—and she, of course, says yes.

RMDS's new location has just opened, the very year Anna was born, thanks to a $13 million grant from the Colorado Department of Education. Once housed in a colorless strip mall, the school now sits on ten wide-open acres in the windy yellow valley tucked between the foothills and the city. As we approach the school on Kipling Street, it's visually noticeable immediately, with an exterior painted in bold stripes and huge letters spelling out RMDS facing east. Architecturally modern, with long windows, steel framing, and a big dreamy playground, the school holds 130 students from preschool through twelfth grade.

When we walk in, I'm struck by the school's openness, its good energy, its *silence.* As we follow the signs for the toddler program, I notice the hallways are super wide—at least twenty feet across—and without lockers. Instead, floor-to-ceiling whiteboards run the length of the walls, and students have scrawled messages to each other on them, drawn murals. I'll find out later that the building was designed by a Deaf architect (with input from the students themselves), and its feel is all intentional: the wide hallways are so students can walk side by side and sign with each other on the way to class. The floors also have a bouncy give to them so that someone who can't hear can feel another person approaching from behind.

At the end of the hallway, we reach the preschool pod where the toddler program is being held behind a wall of glass. Pooled in natural light and the happy gleam of hundreds of children's books, the room contains a handful of instructors and what looks like twenty very young kids. They're on the ground, kneeling over plastic, yarn-filled totes. We stand in the doorway for a few seconds taking in the scene, as the toddlers make "ice cream sundaes" with multicolored yarn pompoms and construction paper cones. The kids are moving with rapid excitement, picking up the poofs with plastic ice cream scoopers and topping them with paper confetti sprinkles. All of them are ages zero to three, they're either deaf or hard of hearing, or they're those children's siblings.

It's a diverse group, in age, in race, and in needs. Some children are in wheelchairs, others on oxygen. One boy there is in a reclined and always accompanied state (due to his having seizures almost constantly, I'll learn), and given his eyes—which are raised to the ceiling and mostly white—and his presence here, I realize he must be deafblind. The teachers are forming words in his hands, bringing the pompoms against the sides of his face so he can feel what the others can see. A few of the children have CHARGE syndrome, a genetic condition that, like CMV, can cause deafness, blindness, balance problems, and developmental delays but is more visible than CMV (though much rarer) because it often presents with unusually shaped ears.

And of course, there are the children with unattributed mobility issues and unexplained hearing loss, whose parents will later tell me, astounded, that they've never heard of congenital CMV.

What I notice most is a boy-girl pair of twins who look like they're about three. The girl has pin-tight strawberry-blond curls covering her ears, where I can just barely make out the glittery processors of her hearing aids. Her brother is a bright-eyed, bright blond-haired boy with a short haircut. He is wearing cochlear implants.

It's the first time I've seen CIs in person, and I catch myself staring from just inside the door. The processors are the same color as his skin, and they blink lime green above each ear. The boy is turning his head quickly, playing passionately in the ice cream tub with all the other kids, and the implants are staying perfectly put. He holds up a carefully balanced cone. He looks toward his dad. Then he smiles, opens his mouth, and *speaks*. I try to swallow the start of tears before anyone sees.

But someone does. A man is making his way toward me. His name tag says Dan, and I assume from his springy hair, which holds the same Christmas-ribbon curls as the girl's, that he's the father of the twins.

"I bet you're overwhelmed, Mom!" he says to me from behind round, wire-frame glasses before I even have time to register that I am. "That's okay," he says, patting me gently on the back. "We'll get you all primed up!"

Then he kneels down to Zaley, asks her how old she is, and his daughter trots over so the two can size each other up. I'm relieved that someone has talked to us, that Zaley might have a friend, that Dan isn't using his hands.

Once I look around, I notice that more of the parents actually seem to be speaking than signing, and I remember something I read: that the majority of deaf children are born to hearing parents. Which means, when I see it at RMDS, that almost all the children in the toddler program have either hearing aids or cochlear implants or another kind of implant called a Baha that transmits sound by way of bone conduction at the back of the ear.

I know that 90 percent of deaf children won't learn sign language because they'll get cochlear implants and their parents will use primarily spoken language. I wonder how many of us here will fit into that statistic, despite this program's mission to provide an ASL foundation to our kids.

A woman in her late forties approaches us next. "Come join the ice cream party!" she says, while signing at the same time. "I'm Susie! I heard you might be coming, and I'm so glad you did!"

Susie looks just like a friend I grew up with, and I love her energy and verve immediately. I can tell Susie loves what she's doing. There are some people who do their jobs, and there are others who embody their jobs, and Susie is clearly the second. Right away she makes a foreign room and a foreign language, for us, a home.

"Get right in there, girl!" Susie urges Zaley, ushering her toward the action and eliminating my fear that this world might exclude Zaley because she can hear. Susie always uses simultaneous communication, or SimCom: using sign language and spoken language at the same time, to make the program accessible for both groups of families and kids—those who sign and those who don't. Next, she and the program coordinator, who is a congenitally deaf and beautiful woman named Steph, distribute take-home laminated cards (Zaley and I love anything laminated), with pictures of a Deaf instructor signing *sprinkles* and *flavor* and *chocolate, vanilla, strawberry*.

And finally, once the yarn activity is over, Steph and Susie reveal the literal cherry on top: the kids all get to make real ice cream sundaes complete with syrup, whipped cream, and maraschinos, and they'll get to *eat them*. One look at Zaley tells me she'll be sold on sign language for life.

———

Before we leave, Dan asks me Anna's level of hearing loss. When I tell him she's profoundly deaf and we're thinking of getting her cochlear implants, he tells me he'll have us over for dinner. "But before then," he adds, "let me show you how these puppies work." Then he beckons and calls to his son: "Austin, come here!"

Austin comes right over, even though the room is loud with the bustle of spoons clinking and babies screaming. "Can I see one of your ears?" Dan asks him. Then Austin reaches up, pulls one of the implants off his head, and hands it to his dad.

"See how it turned orange? That means it's not working now that it's not connected to him." As soon as he puts it back on Austin's head, the light flashes green again.

"So . . . can he hear everything now?" I ask.

"Yep. Watch this!" Then Dan whispers, "Can you hear me?"

And in the chaos of twenty toddlers eating ice cream, Austin whispers back, "Yes."

5

Nonetheless, I hesitate to schedule Anna's cochlear implant surgery. Most of me believes it's the right thing for our family. But part of me also feels like it's unfair—or maybe just not cool—to make her unlike all the wonderful Deaf people we've met and now call friends. And if necessity is the mother of invention, I know it must be the mother of language acquisition, too. If Anna ends up not needing ASL, we probably won't devote ourselves as fully to learning it, and I badly want sign language to be a permanent presence in our lives. I don't just want to learn sign so that Anna has it as a backup for when her implants are broken or when she's in the bath; I feel a summoning on a much deeper level than that.

In a 2015 essay for *The New Yorker,* writer Jhumpa Lahiri writes about her longing to learn Italian, even though she feels that she's in a state of "linguistic exile" from it—she speaks English primarily, and moreover, her mother tongue is Bengali. "Almost as soon as we met," she writes, "Italian and I were separated. My yearning seems foolish. And yet I feel it." I'm surprised when I read this because it's how I've always felt in relationship to ASL, even as a child, before I had a reason to know it. I can still feel its distance from me, and yet I long to call it my own.

Some of our therapists have implied that using sign language might detract from Anna's acquisition of speech. But you can't silence the callings of the heart; nor can you choose the language of those callings. In my heart there will always be a hand opening and closing. It's not just a hand beckoning—though it is that, too. It's a hand that is signing.

Luke reminds me that getting Anna cochlear implants in no way means we can't be a family who uses ASL, too. "I know," I tell him, "but I keep thinking more about my ambivalence than I do about our decision."

"That's because that's the way you are."

He's right. But here's the other problem, the one that's more cultural than personal: while my intention is, no doubt, to give Anna the best chance at a connected life, the problem is that the only image I have of life is the privileged one I have lived. When I picture Anna as culturally Deaf and implant-free, the image isn't nearly as vivid as the vision modern technology and mainstream culture have promised me, where Anna chats with anyone she meets, goes to school anywhere she wants, gets a job because she can speak.

I'm also wary of my decision to get her implants because I generally distrust technology, and I know that using technology with the good intention of making meaningful connections can go royally awry. Look at the history of the telephone, I tell Luke—a device that has connected people more than any other invention in history, but was created by a man who wanted to fix things to such an extent that he foresaw a perfect world as a world without deaf people in it.

Alexander Graham Bell had a deaf mother and a deaf wife, and he devoted much of his life to teaching the deaf to speak. He was also a prolific inventor, and perhaps because of his ability to create devices and objects that solved problems—the metal detector, to locate the bullet lodged inside assassinated President James Garfield; the audiometer, to detect hearing problems; the graphophone, to play long pieces of music in the absence of instruments—he thought of different people, deaf people, as a problem to fix, too. As an early supporter of the eugenics movement (which translates literally as "well-born"), Bell would go on to publicly broadcast his opinion that two congenitally deaf people shouldn't marry because then they'd produce more deaf children—offspring, he believed, who would be "attended by calamitous results." Bell was so against deaf identity, he pursued outlawing sign language and making spoken English the only language that could be used in the United States.

Knowing his story, knowing his goals, I'm especially aware of making sure Anna's cochlear implants are chosen out of thoughtfulness and love, not cultural persuasion, not homogenization.

"Of course they are," Luke says. "You've probably thought this through more than anyone who's ever gotten them. Plus, don't you think she'll still feel different with her cochlear implants?"

My rational husband. Right again.

My defense of Anna's implants is becoming what they call in the church *apologetics*—that is, explaining your beliefs to your critics, which in my experience is really, first, defending yourself to yourself. My first apology: My motives are opposite those of a man who saw a singular language as something so superior as to be made law. In fact, if I could have one superpower, it would be to speak and sign every language in the world. I would give everyone else that superpower, too.

Apology number two: If you think I'm trying to make Anna not-deaf, you should know that I would never take Anna's access to silence away (which is why I'm not a fan of fully implanting cochlear devices inside a deaf person's head—an innovation that may happen during Anna's lifetime). And three: I see cochlear implants not as a cure for deafness, as many people do, but as an additional sensor of the sensory world.

Plus, there are some undoubtedly cool things about CIs: if I clip a small microphone to my collar and Anna wears waterproof sleeves over her implants, she'll eventually be able to hear me ten feet underwater as if I'm standing next to her on land. When she's a little older, we can change her settings to Bluetooth at the push of a button, and the sound from a cellphone or an iPad will go directly into her brain—she'll hear the *Frozen* soundtrack on the way to Alaska, while the person sitting next to her won't hear a note.

I love this irony: that Anna will have a superhero's sense of hearing. Which means, then, that people like A. G. Bell would have to concede that my deaf child's ability to hear the world is, in many ways, superior to those not born deaf.

The difficulty, I guess, is not that I disagree with cochlear implants. I like them, I think they're amazing, and I love the culture of the Deaf community, too. The problem is that I have to make this decision—a decision that will deeply impact the rest of Anna's life, her personality, her language, her friends—without her consent.

Nonetheless, we decide yes to cochlear implants. Yes to two languages. Yes to Anna ever deciding to change her mind.

———

There's one more thing about implants I haven't yet had the courage to face. So one morning I run the Google search I've continued to postpone: *What does it sound like to hear through cochlear implants?*

I'm holding Anna and standing in the kitchen, and Zaley is perched on the counter, watching me type and wondering aloud if she'll get to look at photos of treehouses once I'm done. A few CI videos pop up, and I choose one that looks like it will be less sentimental, more on the scientific side of things: *Cochlear implant: simulation on speech and music,* it reads. I gather whatever grit I have. Then I press the small white triangle in the middle of the screen.

"What are we watching, Mom?" Zaley asks. But there's no movie, just jumping squares to indicate the rising and falling of the volume that has just begun.

"We're going to hear . . . what Anna might hear . . . once she hears," I say, knowing this must mean nothing to Zaley at all. But she sits up straight, and I hold Anna facing out, and we all absorb, in silence, the hypothetical sound of Anna's future.

First comes a raspy, electronic voice repeating a sentence. The noise is more abrasive than I've braced myself for—like heavy sandpaper sliding across a table or, even at its clearest, a garbled, deep, Darth Vader–like drone. The vowels and consonants can barely be differentiated; their tonelessness is offensive, abrupt. I can't even tell what the voice is saying as it repeats itself. Once the simulation is over, the authentic human voice reveals its statement, which is, unbelievably enough: "What kind of bait do you use to catch salmon?"

"Herring!" Zaley exclaims next to me, correctly.

Then starts the simulation of music. I think of how my mom's breath went away when I told her that Anna was deaf. Listening to the cochlear implant version of music does the same air-snatching thing to my chest. I gasp. It sounds like a hundred feet stomping in shallow water. It sounds slashing, dark, and harsh. It is not a song. It is not beautiful. It is not what I want to give Anna when we give her the thing we call music. There is rhythm, yes, but when the track switches to the real flamenco song I can hear, when I feel the pure, trilling elegance of the violin and the irreplaceable pleasure of the tambourine, the lilting strings, the luminous melody, I completely fall apart.

I have to sit down. I lift Zaley off the counter with one arm and push Anna tighter to my heart with the other. I walk stiffly into the family room and sink onto the couch, where Zaley finds a spot on my lap, next to her sister, and stares at me in the terrible quiet my tears create around her. She strokes my hair. She wraps my free fingers into hers. She says, "Mommy, don't cry. Here, let's play with some beads."

⁂

After Zaley goes down for her nap, I pass my computer in the kitchen, and something catches my eye: it's the thumbnail for another YouTube video, recommended because of the video we'd watched. It's a short documentary of a Deaf woman dancing in a ballroom competition.

I push play. She goes to Oxford and has cochlear implants. As the clear sound of the ballroom music replaces the leaden sound of the simulation still banging around in my head, I start to loosen my hold on the pain I'm conjuring into Anna's future—a pain I've imagined will come based on what *I'm* experiencing: a comparison of actual music to electronic projections. It's a comparison Anna will, fortunately, never have to make. She'll hear it one way and one way only—a type of hearing she can either accept or reject.

I think, then, of a statement in a memoir called *Deafness* I'd recently read, written in 1969 by the deaf poet David Wright: "It is the non-deaf who absorb a large part of the impact of the disability," he writes. "The limitations imposed by deafness are often less noticed by its victims than by those with whom they have to do."

I don't like the word *victim,* but I realize he's right—so far I've been the one impacted by Anna's deafness, not Anna. She is none the wiser, a grinning little ogre bemused by any appearance of motion or light. Who am I to own Anna's happiness or her sadness, her experience of sound or music, before they even exist? And if I make Anna's suffering too much my own, I know I run the risk of distorting the great pleasure she will take in life and bring to mine.

The Deaf woman in front of me dances gracefully and on beat. She seems genuinely joyful, saying that dance is where she can "bring music to life." At the end of the video, she takes off her cochlear implants and signs to her friends. Her challenges don't look so different from the challenges I'd faced in my twenties: belonging, loneliness, love, and how to wrap everything up in language.

"Deafness," Wright says, "does not seem to me to be a disproportionate element of the predicament in which I find myself; that is to say the predicament in which we are all involved because we live and breathe."

———

Sometime in December, Luke suggests we set the date for Anna's surgery. In a stroke of crazy serendipity, our insurance says not only that they'll cover it but that we can choose the date ourselves. I'm elated—and totally skeptical that this rare act of bureaucratic mercy could actually be true.

Anna will turn one year old in June. But if we wait till then, as the FDA currently recommends, Luke will already be fishing, and I know I can't face her surgery without him. Our cochlear implant audiologist—a woman named Allison Biever who's tiny, lovable, always heel-clad, and a mother of three teenage girls—says ten months would be ideal. Other countries implant children as early as six months of age, and even in the United States, if a child had meningitis, they would rush the surgery earlier than twelve months, before the ear canal ossifies with bone. These kids do just fine.

At ten months, Anna will be big enough that there won't be as much risk with general anesthetic, and those extra two months of learning are proving to be noticeably beneficial for children implanted under the age of one. We set the date for April 20—two weeks before the start of fishing season. And our insurance sends a letter approving it, which feels like I've just opened a golden ticket in the mail.

6

The night before Anna's procedure, I try to do as little mental preparing and as much logistical preparing as possible. If I think too much about the puffy sack that will do the work of Anna's lungs, I can feel a downward rush of panic from my shoulders to my hips. Instead, I clip each of Anna's fingernails and toenails before I place her in the bath. At ten months old, when other babies her age are pulling themselves up on furniture, even taking their first steps, she's just starting to have enough core and neck strength to sit up with my hand behind her back.

But in the bath, she likes to lie down in a few inches of bubbly water and gaze up at my face. I cup her head in one hand, then rub shampoo into her ever-lightening hair. I wash between each of her fingers, beneath her fatless chin, around her outie belly button that's shaped like a mini M&M. Underwater, I massage behind each ear where the surgeon will slide a knife before he drills out her mastoid bone and inserts a magnet, a receiver, and a long strip of sensors.

I look at her head one last time with its sudsy hair and lack of devices. Like every mother gazing at their child at this age, in a moment of peace, part of me doesn't want her to change, ever. She's always alert and practically motionless in the tub, made careful by the surrounding pressure of the water. When I lift her from the bubbles, she melts against me with a sigh of trust. She's the size of a three-month-old. She smells like a Creamsicle.

In the hospital bag, I pack a zip-up onesie that I won't have to lift over her bandage-wrapped head. A soft blanket. A bottle she won't take. A book I won't read. Really, there is no preparing to do. This is just my nature: I make lists to make waiting seem less passive. I know

I can't prepare Anna for hearing any more than I'd been prepared for her deafness.

———

Anna is not allowed to eat anything eight hours prior to surgery. So the morning of her procedure, when I have to wake her in the dark and deprive her of her routine morning feed, I'm afraid the day will start with her upset. But she looks straight at me in the glow of the nightlight, silent, smiling, and angelically content. In my head is Psalm 57 on repeat: *"My heart is ready, O God; my heart is ready, And I will sing!"*

Luke knows I won't be able to eat either, so he has my coffee ready downstairs, and he says he'll drive. I put Anna in her car seat, and we ride to Swedish Hospital in the most significant silence I've ever experienced (which is only possible because Zaley is with my parents). It's dawn—my favorite time of day, the time of day Anna was born—and the flush of light over the eastern plains gradually turns the mountains from a midnight blue to a backlit maroon. As the sun inflames the western range, I think of how transformed Anna will soon be, too, and yet like that mountain, she'll still be the same entity, composed of the same elemental beauty.

This might seem like an exaggeration, but there is life saving and life *altering,* and I can't think of something more momentous happening to a person than cochlear implant surgery. I know surgeries like heart transplants are longer and much more involved, but the heart that has always been beating will continue, post-op, to do its same function, which is imperceptibly beat. The body does not feel, in an indelible instant, the addition of a component that never was. With cochlear implants, a brain that has never processed sound will "hear" it in one pathway-carving, split-second moment, nine days after her surgery, when we'll sit in Allison's office for Anna's "activation day."

Anxious as I am, I also can't resist the preemptory joy I take in knowing that what was once unknown to Anna will soon be irrevocably known. Voices, verses, music, wind. Noisemakers, sizzling, shouting, laughter.

I can't wait to read to her. To whisper to her. To see her light up, as I did, to the first sound of her father's voice.

The staff at Swedish is kind, patient, and excited for us as they slip a puppy-covered gown onto Anna's narrow frame. The nurse hands me a pair of scrubs and pulls the curtain closed with a clatter of the overhead rings. Sounds seem magnified, profound. Luke says goodbye to us, and as I follow the surgeon, Dr. Kelsall, to the silver doors, Anna's life, her silence, flashes before my eyes. I wish Anna would look at me and give me some sign that yes, this *optional* surgery is what she would want, too. But she's just herself—content again and watching the metal doors open to let us in.

I've never been so scared in my life. The pre-op room is bright white, and nine or ten people are standing there, hands arranged in all the ways of waiting—folded, crossed at their middles, on their hips—all of them ready to attend to Anna, my treasure. She seems so important, the center of everything, and I'm moved to tears by this reverence that mirrors my own. The air and the light feel sharp and tangible, as though they're sundering my skin, and I think of something my friend Lizzy said one breezy day when we were walking with our daughters: "It's like when you have kids, the wind isn't just the wind anymore. Everything slices you open to a greater degree."

Lizzy was right. The wind isn't just the wind. The oxygen mask isn't just an oxygen mask. This is my tiny daughter underneath it, puffing wet breaths into the clear, soft cup. Her violet eyelids closing, her white arms going limp.

"Perfect job," Dr. Kelsall says, putting his hand on my shoulder. "She didn't fight the anesthesia at all. She's going to do great. We'll keep you posted."

As I walk out of the room on legs that don't feel like my own, I think of all the other CMV mothers who've had to leave their children on the gurney repeatedly, moms whose kids have needed brain surgeries, back fusions, hip dysplasia osteotomies. I feel it in a weakening flood, how heartbreaking this place is—this liminal space where we are separated from our children, having to make the choices their bodies couldn't make for themselves.

I think of something a CMV doctor, Martha Yow, wrote almost

twenty years ago, in 1992. She'd calculated that in the twenty years that had elapsed since Thomas Weller's CMV article appeared in *The New England Journal of Medicine* in 1971, approximately 170,000 children in the United States had developed deafness and neurological impairment due to CMV. "We should not wait another 20 years," she insisted, "while thousands of additional children are born seriously handicapped."

Those twenty years have already happened. Our children have already been born. Here I am waiting for mine to wake up, incisions behind her ears a sign of intervening, a marker of our loving, but also, a lifelong reminder of congenital CMV.

———

Luke wraps me in his strong arms in the waiting area and tells me to take some deep breaths, and after about two breaths I forget I'm supposed to do that. Then my phone rings. It's my childhood friend Carol, who has already given me one of the most loving gestures I've ever received from a friend: along with Karen—who took care of the horses with me—they've been taking evening ASL classes ever since we found out that Anna is deaf. Carol is outside the hospital now with breakfast sandwiches. We meet her in the horseshoe-shaped driveway, and when she asks how I'm doing, I cave and sob. I feel miles away from Anna even though she's just upstairs, and I rush back to where she and I can be on the same floor.

Even though I thought I'd be too nervous to eat, I'm ravenous and eat my sandwich in the waiting room, in a blue leather seat. But I can't talk. Or read. I think of praying, and I remember what my brother David once told me about prayer: that it exists outside of time—that you can pray for things that have already happened. I don't know where Dr. Kelsall is in Anna's surgery—if he has broken through her skin, if the first magnet is already set in its perpetual place. But if what David said is true, it doesn't matter how much of the surgery is left. It doesn't actually matter if I'm praying for the Anna that had been in my womb or the Anna who's in the operating room. In the clinical chair where so many mothers have waited with more worry than anywhere else in their lives, I land on the simplest, most steadying prayer I can find, a line from Exodus 14: "The Lord your God will fight for you, and you need only sit still."

———

Two and a half hours later, the nurse enters the waiting room. Because we've been prepared that some bilateral CI surgeries can last upward of six hours, I'm sure something must be wrong.

But no—the nurse is smiling. "Anna is done," she says. "She did beautifully. You can come back."

A few young nurses are tending to Anna in the recovery room, and they turn to us when we enter the whispering space. They're cooing over how cute she is; they tell me she's doing just great. One of them hands Anna to me in her too-big dog gown, and I can tell she's fine, but I can also tell she's in pain. My heart careens toward hers, and yet at the same time, I feel a shrinking back, a shame, a self-questioning, knowing that we created the condition from which she'll need to recover.

I press her against me and sit down in the recliner, and she buries her head in my chest. Her IV-punctured hand is wrapped up in a mitt of gauze, and unlike the clean white bandages I'd seen online of kids who'd gone through the same surgery, hers are the real thing, not the changed dressings appropriate for posting to the public. Her mitten is red-brown with blood, and above her searching eyes, so is her crown of gauze. I gaze down at her on my chest and I say, weeping, "I'm sorry baby, I'm so sorry."

———

The next day is rough. No matter what I do to comfort her, Anna groans all day, on and off. She bleeds from her ears and her nose. The skin surrounding her eyes takes on a swollen, ocean-colored hue. The bandage is wrapped around her head like an American Gladiator helmet, and because it's pushing down on her eyebrows, she glares at us from under the dressings all day as if she resents what we did.

At dusk, Luke and I take a long walk around our neighborhood with Anna in the baby carrier below my chin. As I cup both sides of Anna's head in my hands, I can feel the raised, quarter-size ridges of the magnets under her skin, the cresting of our lives toward a totally uncharted shore. Back at the house, I try to comfort her by pushing her on the porch swing in the mild spring breeze, but even there, in her favorite spot, she looks upset. At night, she sleeps upright, on my stomach, like a small injured animal. It's one of the most crushing days I've ever had as a mother; I feel that I have strong-armed her into a pain whose redemption is by no means guaranteed.

Mercifully, though, by the end of the second day, just as Dr. Kelsall had said, she seems to have almost fully healed. Her sleep is back to normal, and she doesn't even need Tylenol. She also doesn't seem to notice that there's anything new inside her head.

But her ears! The surgeon's office had failed to mention that once the bandage was off, her ears would stick straight out from her head at almost ninety degrees. I'm horrified when we unwrap the gauze and her ears don't float back down to their natural, tucked-back place. I take pictures of her, then compare them to pictures of her before the surgery to make sure my eyes aren't playing tricks.

"Luke!" I cry. "This can't be right! What if they sewed them back on wrong?"

"They'll go down," he says, unflappable as ever and anger-inducingly calm. "We can call the doctor if you're really worried."

When I do, the nurse says, "Oh yeah. That happens. It can take a few weeks for them to go back down."

7
———

Then it's the day my deaf daughter might hear.

Karen takes Zaley to the museum for the morning, and Luke and I meet our parents at Swedish Hospital at ten a.m. An indoor bridge connects the parking garage to the audiology clinic, and as we cross it, its significance isn't lost on me: the next time we walk across, in the opposite direction, Anna will be spanning two worlds, the hearing and the deaf.

In Allison's small, packed office, the grandparents sit upright on chairs against a wall of windows. Luke and I sit next to Allison's desk. Luke holds Anna in a magenta headband facing outward in his lap, and I sit next to them, holding her hand.

I know I should be thrilled, but I feel disheveled and overwhelmed. I wish I'd washed my hair, wasn't wearing what I am. I look out the window, at the snow sweeping upward and sideways in the smoke-puffed sky outside the hospital, and I feel as all-directional and detached as that snow. I'm also nauseous that these things, once activated, won't work; that maybe our parents have come all this way to see nothing; or that my child will hate the sound of sound.

Allison is seated at her desk in a black dress and black heels. She swivels her chair to face us as we all wait, on edge.

"Anyone have any questions," she asks, "before we begin?"

Luke and I shake our heads, so very ready to proceed with the event, but already my dad is asking Allison about remote programming and replacement parts and the shelf-life of the implant, till my mom whispers, "Jerry!" so we can move on. Allison smiles patiently, waiting for any last questions, then tells us what to expect.

"Anna might look up or smile. Or she might start crying," she cautions cheerfully, attempting to protect us from our inevitable expectations. "Or we might not see any reaction at all. And those are all normal reactions."

She says that once she connects the battery to the implant, the processor will need a few seconds before it transmits any sound.

"I'll count to three. You ready?" she asks Luke and me.

We nod.

Then she twists the battery onto the processor hanging off of Anna's right ear.

"One . . . two . . . three," she says. And then it happens: "Now it's on. Anna . . . can you hear me?"

Anna's neck goes rigid, and she looks straight ahead. She looks stunned. All air, verbs, nouns, sounds flee the room.

Then, "Hi," I say, tentative, not at all what I'd planned. "Hi, baby! Hi!"

Anna's body slinks back. Her hands reach for me, for Luke, for protection from this shocking shift, from whatever this is.

There's no doubt about it: our deaf daughter is hearing.

———

On the bridge back to the car, while both of Anna's implants are channeling sound into her brain, I place her on the thick windowsill, and she presses her palms and nose against the glass. I lean close to her ears and say what I've been wanting her to hear since she was born: "I love you, Anna. I love you, I love you." I can't tell if she turns to reach for me because she heard me or because I am her everything.

In the multilevel parking lot, which echoes like a tunnel, our parents wipe their eyes and congratulate us. But Anna, quiet as ever, just watches the snow. Allison has warned us this might happen— that we might think the whole thing was a fluke, that her ears don't work—but this has not prepared me for the validation I crave. I want to see, right now, that this was worth the risk, the time, the pain. When I push the round button and the elevator arrives with a chime, Anna's head doesn't turn, doesn't seek the source, doesn't change. In the car, I take the implants off her, as instructed, so she doesn't detach them, put them in her mouth, and choke.

When we get to Karen's apartment, I kneel down and tell Zaley what has happened, but she's more interested in saying goodbye to Karen's cat than in understanding the gravity of Anna's greatest change. Subtly, almost imperceptibly, Karen signs *I love you* to Anna as we're walking out the door.

———

When we get home around noon, the reality of the morning starts to seep in. While I'd pictured peacefully entering our new existence, Zaley has other plans. In the family room, before I've even taken Anna out of her car seat, Zaley is sprinting laps around the coffee table, stopping only to give me a crazed look before slamming, stomach first, into the couch. And it's unusually dark. The weight of the wet spring snow has bent the branches of the cherry blossom tree next to the window in our backyard, and the family room appears darkened by a canopy of ashen pink blooms. The light in the room is unlike the light that usually fills it, and I feel the same shading of my heart as the gray that has seeped over the walls.

I sit down on the couch, unbuckle Anna from her seat, and place her on my lap, facing out. Then I take the $25,000 beige devices out of their shiny black case, and I slide the magnets and processors back onto her head. The lights turn green. I say something to her, but she doesn't even shift. *The world was supposed to be changed,* I think, looking out at the drooped and dripping tree. Instead, it seems like winter has come again.

All the ensuing years appear before me: the hundreds of times every week we will attach, lose, search for, and reattach her implants. The imperative is now on me that I never felt with her hearing aids: these devices are real, and she really needs them. This is a responsibility I somehow overlooked in the days leading up to her surgery: Anna's ability to hear depends upon my ability to make her cochlear implants available for her, every moment, every day. The kids who are able to speak wear them for at least eight hours daily, which is quadruple how long she ever left her hearing aids on her head.

I hold Anna in my arms and wonder, again, if I'll see anything that indicates we did the right thing. Without looking at me, she pulls the implants out with both hands and throws them onto the floor.

———

Every other day for the next two weeks, we up the amplitude of Anna's implants with a skinny remote I carry around in my purse when Zaley isn't trying to pretend it's her phone. The amplitude is not simply volume; it's a specific setting for each ear, similar to a prescription for eyeglasses, where each side is programmed to meet her brain's needs. We know the setting because Allison can plug a cord into Anna's implant that leads to the computer, and on the screen, we can see her neural response telemetry—basically, the specific frequencies she needs to make out every tone, crisp and true, on the musical scale and in speech. This process is called MAPping the implants, a term I love. It's like every time we go in, Allison adds to Anna's internal atlas—her brain a compass directing her ears.

At one point, I asked Allison if we should continue going to Alaska when it might best serve Anna to be home, where Allison could adjust her settings in person, as needed. But it turns out, remote programming is standard practice for audiologists and auditory-verbal therapists; rural deaf children can't commute into the office every month or every week.

It turns out, too, that Allison is Canadian and grew up at exactly the same latitude as Sitka. She prefers cool summers and tons of green over ninety-degree, wildfire-inducing heat. She doesn't see any need for us to make an Alaskan exit due to Anna's needs. She has a tablet she can send to Alaska with me every summer, through which she'll be able to adjust Anna's MAP no matter the fog, the distance, or the dense forest of our daughter's developing brain.

———

After a few heartsick weeks of wondering if we've made the wrong choice, Anna's changes suddenly appear. Watching her hearing come alive is the kind of walloping thrill I'd wish for every parent to experience in life. If I say hi but I don't lift my hand, she waves from having *heard me,* her hand slowly opening and closing "like a small starfish," my brother David says. Zaley hides inside cabinets, calls out "Anna," and Anna bursts into a smile. My still-deaf child, lighting up at the sound of her name!

And we marvel at Anna in her silence, too. When her ears are off and Zaley shakes her long blond bangs in Anna's face like a rabid dog, Anna giggles till her eyes close and she falls over on her side. I love that her sense of humor has nothing to do with her sense of hearing.

It's like we've activated an on switch in Anna herself. Even though she's still toothless, she's eating pea-size bites of elk burger and salmon and blueberries by the half-carton. She can sit up at the table in a high chair, with supports clipped across her chest. She claps when I clap. My brother Michael comes over and plays a playlist he made just for her, and she listens with eyes wide, transfixed. She's laughing more than ever. She sounds like a Tickle Me Elmo. Zaley loves her so much, she shakes her own fists at her sides in restraint and says she wishes she could eat her.

———

For much of Anna's development, I realize, I've been doing subconscious subtraction and addition to her age in my head, as people do for a while when they have a child born premature: *Yes, she's ten months old, but she's more like five months because of congenital CMV. She's ten months old, but she might not have teeth till she's two.* I've been sensitive to—and pained by—Anna's many "ages" since her birth.

The cochlear implants have added a new dimension to this sliding back and forth in time because people refer to Activation Day as a deaf child's "hearing birthday" and say things like *She's one year old, but only two months hearing.* I can barely keep track.

After Anna's activation, I'm ready to get rid of these ableist equations. My friend Beth, whose son has autism, suggests we try a special kind of physical therapy called the Anat Baniel Method, or ABM, which also rejects the idea that all children should be held accountable to a typical timeline. Anat, an Israeli movement therapist, developed the method, cautioning against the damage caused by the "fixing paradigm" in therapy and medicine, and suggested that children who develop differently are not objects to be fixed but works in progress to whom we can pay close attention and deeply connect. ABM works to awaken the neurodiverse brain with variation as opposed to repetition—repetition being the cornerstone of traditional PT.

I love the premise that the brain changes best through creativity, and I love our therapists, Barbara and Andrew—Barbara who has an older child who doesn't speak, and Andrew who worked in Alaska in his twenties. Andrew says that when he first heard of ABM, which was originally created for children who have cerebral palsy or traumatic brain injuries, he thought it was the most humane thing a person could ever do.

At Anna's appointments, they stand back and watch her for minutes on end. Then they lightly tweak what she's doing, tilting her pelvis so she'll learn to strengthen her neck, touching her on her cheek to widen her weaker right eye. If Anna cries at all, the session is over, and I'm to nurse her, then return the next week.

And their excitement about her makes me so excited, too. One day she turns the page of a book! Another day, she reaches out her arm when I hold up her sleeve! And shortly after her activation, Anna sits up for two seconds totally unassisted, and I want to run down the streets, clicking my heels in the air, like someone out of *Oliver Twist*. I decide I'll never subtract from where Anna is, in her moment, again.

———

To get the boat into the water, haul the totes out of storage, and stretch sheets over the beds, Luke heads to Alaska a few weeks before us. And so one weekend, I bring the girls down to my parents' house where I'm able, in so many ways, to revert to the child I was. I eat cereal anytime I want. I sit on the back porch with my mom and Zaley, watching the sun dapple the twin apple trees where I once broke my wrist. My dad pushes Zaley in the swing, my mom makes iced tea, and my parents and I delight in the things I might otherwise miss in my kids. Without my mom and dad, I know I would enjoy motherhood half as much as I do.

One night, with Anna next to me in my childhood bed, it's the middle of the night when something wakes me up. I sit up and listen. Outside the window, two owls are calling to each other in the dark. I know there are two because the first owl keeps getting interrupted by the second owl's higher-pitched hoot.

There's a floodplain at the edge of my parents' neighborhood that harbors wilder animals than you might expect in the suburbs: coyotes and foxes, bobcats and owls and hawks. I've always loved their nocturnal calls. They sound like longing and sorrow, but also like parents announcing the protection of their young.

I wonder if Anna can hear the owls. Then I remember, she doesn't have her implants on, and she is deaf. I want to tell her about their sound. I want to tell her about her silence. Years later, I do.

PART IV

PLEASURE

"The things that we love tell us what we are."

SAINT THOMAS AQUINAS

With Anna's surgery behind us and hope in front of us, I feel like I'll be able to handle her diagnosis this summer in Alaska. And I can. We are going on with our lives, because what else do you do? There is milk to be poured and avocados to be smashed on toast, and out the back window, the gillnetters are nudging out beyond the safety of the sound. Zaley has made a nest behind the couch with clean laundry so she can reenact *Are You My Mother?* with herself cast as the mother and Anna as the baby bird.

And so things are feeling fairly stable, until I turn on the news.

———

I'm picking Anna's implant off the floor when I hear an Anchorage newscaster's grave warning about another congenital disease. It's a virus, too, though it's actually nowhere near Alaska or most of the Lower 48. The Zika virus, the broadcaster says, spreads through mosquitoes, can cause birth defects, and is preventable through behavioral change. If contracted congenitally, Zika can cause microcephaly, vision issues, and Guillain-Barré Syndrome, or GBS—a long-term autoimmune disease often set in motion by an infection that can render the body weakened, tingling, paralyzed in severe cases, and riddled with pain.

Remembering that CMV can cause GBS, I go to the Mayo Clinic website, which explains that Guillain-Barré can be caused by a stomach or respiratory illness, or—they've recently added—the Zika virus. But predictably, there's no mention of CMV. This is despite the fact that CMV—and not just congenital CMV but also the plain old CMV that any child or adult can catch—is actually the most common viral trigger of Guillain-Barré. I wonder how many other autoimmune diseases are never connected to an infection with CMV.

We only get a few channels on the old-fashioned rabbit ears I've rigged with aluminum foil behind the TV, so I switch from the local Anchorage news to the *Today* show, where they too are talking about Zika. On the screen, they show six pictures in a grid: all the babies have severe microcephaly, with their heads not just small but also flat on top, and they're all dark-skinned. Online, I see the same visual trend. It looks like a place and a disease we can stay away from, if we choose. And this is what the media is encouraging us to do: if we stay away from the unfortunates near our borders, we won't have babies like them.

On my computer, I also read that the Obama administration is seeking $1.9 billion in emergency funding to prophylactically control Zika's impact on Americans through vaccine development, mosquito-controlling technologies, and pregnancy monitoring programs , even though I know that the Institute of Medicine has declared CMV the number-one priority in the world for vaccine development since the year 2000. If Zika is surging out of control, I wonder if it's going to oust CMV from this designated—though underacknowledged—spot?

My worry blazes into anger when I go to CDC.gov and see there's nothing like a surge: there haven't been *any* documented cases of congenital Zika disease in the United States.

I'm reattaching Anna's implant to her head—an intervention set into motion by a far more rampant, homegrown American virus no one knows about—when I actually have to sit down because of what I hear next: a man named Anthony Fauci is admitting that the federal government is being forced to shift money from other diseases to finance a disease that barely exists in the United States. Namely, money is being transferred away from Ebola, cancer, diabetes, heart disease, and mental health. Fauci doesn't mention CMV by name because, I figure, there's no money to be taken from CMV.

When I go to the website for the National Institute of Allergy and Infectious Diseases, which Fauci directs, I find CMV is nowhere in sight—it's not listed under "Diseases and Conditions" in general, and it's not listed in the more specific category of "Infectious Diseases" alongside things like *leishmaniasis* and *prion disease*, which are incredibly rare in the United States.

I wonder if it's possible that our public health agencies are controlled not necessarily by solid science but by public concern and fear. Later, when I reach out to a scientist at the CDC, he essentially confirms this hunch: "Mostly Congress says, 'we want you to work on this, and here's the money to do it.'" And he explains further, "Because the CDC is a government agency, we can't lobby Congress for money for a certain disease."

Congress, of course, is not made up of doctors or scientists. It's made up of people who listen to people who read the news and watch TV. My assumption is correct: there has never been any money at the CDC earmarked for congenital CMV.

Soon there will be Zika-based graphics, links, registries, tracking programs, and—most painfully for mothers like me—a clickable tab on the CDC site that says, "If Your Family Has Been Affected: Supporting Babies Affected by Zika." Already, the CDC has 750 staff working full time on Zika, even though by the end of the Zika "outbreak" in the United States in 2017, fewer than three hundred babies *total* will have been impacted by a Zika infection. (I don't know the exact number because the CDC removed the webpage that once tracked how many babies here were Zika-affected, congenitally.) The low number isn't because we prevented Zika through effective messaging or a vaccine; it's likely, in part, because enough people in Latin and South America caught Zika for herd immunity to stop its spread.

With CMV's many strains, natural herd immunity isn't possible; you'd need a vaccine for about 60 percent of the population to eradicate the disease. And I read online that the companies trying to make a CMV vaccine haven't finished it yet. For now, as Dr. Gail Demmler-Harrison puts it, the best way to prevent CMV is through the "information vaccine": knowledge that CMV exists.

———

"What is Zika?" Zaley asks from behind the couch. "And why does everyone keep talking about it?" A second later, *Are You My Mother?* comes sailing over the furniture, since she's finished with it now. I look at it on the floor and think about her second question.

It occurs to me that we become involved with diseases the same way we become attached to books. If I were to start reading *Are You My Mother?* on page ten, Zaley probably wouldn't pay much attention. We like to start stories at the beginning. And Zika (though it's actually been around for centuries) *feels* like it's just starting, like we're beginning on the first page of the story. This, of course, is how COVID-19 will feel, too. We are interested, in part, because we witness the plot unravel daily, because we are the characters, and because we participate in the suspense of the narrative—whether it will arrive in the United States, whether we'll contract it, whether we'll stop it.

CMV, on the other hand, has never had a current-day surge; it has always existed, has always infected the same number of children, year in and year out. There's no question about its speed, or its growing severity, or when it will arrive.

CMV is *endemic*, which means it can be regularly found among people. But you'd have to argue your point if you called it an *epidemic*, which, by common definition, contains a component of seasonality: an epidemic is "a widespread occurrence of an infectious disease in a community *at a particular time*." If Zika is like mud left on the floor by someone who has just come in, CMV is like dust.

So whenever someone says to me, "I've heard of Zika, but not CMV," I know that they don't just mean they've *heard* of Zika; they mean they've *seen* it.

And we don't fight a disease unless we can picture what it does.

———

Sociologists have a term for this trick of the brain to take an image and ascribe to it both an importance and an irrational belief that it will happen to us: it's called the availability bias. In her book *Small Animals: Parenthood in the Age of Fear,* journalist and mother Kimberly Brooks explains: "In its simplest terms, the availability [bias] tells us that people judge the likelihood of something happening not by facts or statistics or rational thought, but by the ease with which we can recall an example of its happening."

In other words, if a striking image is available, again and again, we ascribe it prevalence and potency. No matter its smallness in reality, our fear and our impressionable memories transform it into an outsize concern.

The problem, according to Brooks, is not our fear itself. "Concern for one's offspring," she writes, "seems as integral a part of what it means to be human as to live in groups or to look for food and shelter." The crisis is the blindness to truth that can be caused by a sensationalizing, repetitive media that stokes unsubstantiated fear. "One doesn't have to look hard or long," she writes, "to see that parental fears do not always correspond to the most apparent and pressing dangers children face."

Zika isn't the first—or the last—time CMV will been sidelined by a more publicized disease. CMV didn't receive adequate attention or funding at the time of the AIDS crisis in the 1980s either, even though it made a major contribution to mortality in AIDS patients. Dr. Paul Griffiths called this failure to acknowledge and study CMV "unacceptable."

And six years after Anna is born, when hundreds of thousands of Americans are dying in the ICU with COVID-19, a study will conclude that a third of ICU patients will reactivate a latent infection with CMV, which doubles a person's mortality rate.

In *Small Animals,* Kimberly Brooks agrees with the wisdom of sociologist Joel Best: "The people in every era make the same assumption, that they correctly understand the nature of their society's problems."

———

While I'm watching the reels of Zika, I feel the tragedy of the disease, but I have to admit an ugly jealousy, too. I want the photographers to be in some room in Tampa or Boise or Des Moines with a CMV mom. I want to see the graphics for CMV prevention instead of a mosquito's proboscis lancing the skin. And I can see that when the media perpetuates an epidemic of fear by choosing to show only the most severely affected children with any one thing, they don't solve any problems in public health. They fortify a culture in which we are further divided, further convinced and further mistaken that this couldn't possibly be us.

2

———

One thing I thought I would lose when I became a mother was the time I had to read. I feared this loss and gorged on literature in Alaska all summer leading up to Zaley's birth in September 2012. I read more books more quickly than I ever had in my life. That season we lived under Derek and Jules, in a walkout basement with a tribal print futon couch and pipes that banged loudly inside wood-paneled walls when the heat came on. I read in the mornings on that rock-hard couch, surrounded by the sound of clanging metal, till the library opened at ten, and then I settled into one of the reading chairs facing the lighthouse and the sea. I read novels and memoirs, biographies and parenting books that took place in other countries. Because I was visibly pregnant, people would see me reading at the library and they'd gesture, kindly and knowingly, at the book resting on my belly, and they'd whisper things like "You'd better enjoy it while you can!"

This phrase filled me with dread. I knew it was meant to prepare me for what others already knew—how much parenting can consume you—but instead, it consumed me with a worry I didn't end up finding to be true: that parenting would take away the life of my mind.

Of course, after I had Zaley, I was shocked by the soullessness and brain-robbery of sleep deprivation, but this was temporary: within a few weeks, I was delighted to find that—though still low on sleep—I had hours of the day when I could read. While Zaley nursed to sleep, I kept a book in my right hand and turned the pages with the delicacy of a surgeon. (She seemed to wake more easily to the high-pitched crackle of a turning page than to Luke blasting the blender in the kitchen.) Luke was working from home that winter on some business consulting jobs, and he'd appear every hour or so to offer me coffee, or a smoothie, or a break from the baby. I usually took the drinks and kept Zaley with me.

I loved to read with the warmth of her across me, loved this reclamation of my life as both a reader and a mother after I'd been assured I'd lose the former. And I loved the narrators who delved into their subjects with equal parts research and heart.

———

The feeling that my maternal brain was no longer fit for intellectual understanding began during pregnancy. The first ultrasound we'd had for Zaley, when I was eight weeks pregnant, was at a large obstetrical practice connected to Rose Hospital, in central Denver. Luke and I, pregnant with our first child, had arrived both giddy and terrified to see the shape of our progeny on the screen. But when we walked into the ultrasound room, the sonographer was curt and rushed. She was an older woman whose features I don't remember. It's what she said that I'll remember forever.

When she'd located the fetus in my uterus, when our little blueberry was on the screen, heart flashing and body ashudder with blood, she said, "Remember, it's not a baby yet. This is not a baby."

I know some people might not have wanted to be pregnant. But she needed only look at our faces, our gestures, to know that we wanted a child—or she simply could have asked. Maybe she wanted to protect us from potential loss or the projection of our hope. I was, like most pregnant women, well aware of both. I knew there was a one-in-five chance I could miscarry. I knew I'd have the option to run genetic tests. I knew if I found something unexpected, I'd be given the option to have an abortion if I wished.

And yet the other option—the one where I could love unconditionally the seed expanding within me—seemed to be considered ridiculous.

Don't let your emotions get the best of you, the sonographer seemed to be saying, as though "pregnancy brain" had already taken hold, had made me some hormone-driven fool who didn't understand what was happening inside me. And yet neither would the clinic educate me.

A few minutes later, when I met one of the OBs, she wanted to talk about the past and the future, but not what was happening right then. Had I ever contracted an STD? Would we be doing the twelve-week testing? Did we want a handout that explained the cost of the technology that could tell us if our child had trisomy 21? Without my answer, she handed me a shiny brochure with a picture of a happy couple on its cover—people hoping for a baby without whatever diseases would be screened. I wasn't sure if trisomy 21 was Down syndrome or something else. (It is, in fact, Down syndrome.) I wished the cover had shown a child with the diagnosed condition being loved by her parents. But I was never asked to share my feelings. The OB said we should consider paying the private testing company $300.

It felt like my body could make a profit for others, while what I wanted most to know was free, just not freely given: I wanted to know what my body was currently doing. And not the simple, surface-level, hairstyled stuff I could find on pregnancy websites regarding nausea and fatigue. I wanted the nitty-gritty, biological details that seem missing from every woman's understanding of pregnancy.

Not knowing then that insurers don't reimburse physicians as much for the time they spend talking as they do for performing tests and interventions, I longed to know the things I had to learn for myself during subsequent pregnancies: That during pregnancy, the uterus can grow up to five hundred times its original size. That the body nearly doubles its blood volume, and the mother's heart physically increases in weight. That our brains delete gray matter to free up space to focus on a new child. That we produce oxytocin and dopamine to increase the odds that we find our newborn rewarding, no matter what. That pregnancy and motherhood are harder than hell on some women, and easier on others, and I had no guarantee.

Instead, I was given a list of incredibly rare things I should fear. There seemed to be no middle ground between anxiety and complacency, no option for me to be both supportively empowered and appropriately prepared.

The take-home paperwork was a thick packet listing things

like HIV, gonorrhea, chlamydia, hepatitis B, hepatitis C, syphilis, rubella, cystic fibrosis, spinal muscular atrophy, and fragile X syndrome (congenital CMV is actually more common than all of the above *combined*). It cautioned against drinking any alcohol at all during pregnancy, though I would later find out that an occasional drink—even one to two per week, during any trimester—had no consequences on a pregnancy or on children studied years after birth.

The first chapter of my pregnancy contained terse chapters, narrated by joyless guides, who had neither an understanding of their audience nor an awareness that many of the diseases they worried me about were thousands of times less likely than the one I could've learned to prevent.

———

Friends are texting me. They know I know about congenital disease, and they want to know where mosquitoes carrying Zika might find them and make their babies look like the ones they've seen on the news. I would probably do the same, and yet the irony remains: my friends are asking me how best to not have a baby with microcephaly or delays—a baby like mine.

This is a paradox I face intimately on June 17. I'm finishing my coffee at the kitchen island when my phone shifts sideways on the counter. It's a text from my brother Michael. I assume he, too, is wondering about the Zika virus since his wife, Brenda, is due to have their first child in July.

But no: they're on their way to the hospital. She's in labor four weeks early.

My heart speeds in my chest. I know what they might not: preterm labor can be caused by CMV.

———

Michael and Brenda have been incredibly careful throughout her pregnancy, as people with infertility can be. Brenda has severe PCOS—polycystic ovarian syndrome—where cysts form in the ovaries and can prevent pregnancy. Due to PCOS, her ovaries were double the size of what they should have been. After three years of trying to conceive, Brenda and Michael were urged by doctors and acquaintances to consider IVF. But Brenda, a biologist by trade, felt that her obstetrician wasn't looking at the underlying problem, so she switched to a smaller obstetrical practice and found out her infertility was due to her body's dysregulated reaction to insulin.

She went on a hyperstrict diet and lost twenty pounds, but still, she couldn't get pregnant. Her OB then recommended a procedure that many people with PCOS don't know exists; informally known as "the wedge", he would cut a large triangle out of her cyst-covered ovary so it could grow back, fresh. Brenda said yes, and three months after the surgery, she was pregnant.

That was the month we returned from Alaska, with our toddler and our four-month-old daughter who were both likely contagious with CMV.

Michael and Brenda knew how to mitigate their risk of contracting CMV, and they handled it like I picture all people can: it became second nature for them to use what doctors call "universal precautions"—basically, good hygiene to avoid the transmission of fluids. But I feared them coming over anyway; I felt like if anything happened, it would be my fault. Anytime they were on their way, I would race around the house, removing toys and spoons from rooms where Anna or Zaley might have had them in their mouths. I probably didn't need to be so vigilant, since it wasn't like Brenda would be sucking on toys. But they had tried so hard, and it made sense to be extra careful, and so we were.

But here it is June, too early for delivery, and it's my fear—not theirs—standing before me: maybe we have caused someone else's child's disabilities.

When I go to text Michael back, my texts aren't working, and I get the red exclamation mark on my phone that makes my heart rate rise. I call Luke, who's amazingly still in range, and he says, "Keep trying. Turn your phone off and back on."

"I don't have time for that!" I tell him, like I'm a paramedic trying to get them to the hospital or something. Why am I texting anyway? I call my mom. They're admitting Brenda to the hospital now.

My morning takes over: we need groceries; there's a blowout to be changed; Zaley can't find a dress that won't drag in the rain. Then when I park at the grocery store, I go to call my mom again, and my phone isn't working at all.

I'm sitting in front of Lakeside, the rain whipping the windows of our Suburban—the setting of so many revelations in our Alaskan life—when I call Verizon to explain why I really, really need my phone to work today. For the first time in maybe my entire life, the employee on the other end of the line tells me exactly which settings to adjust—and it works!

My phone dings one, two, three times: It's Michael. Brenda just had a baby! It's a girl! Her name is Adelaide, they're going to call her Addie, and—praise the Lord—she weighs seven whole pounds!

There's a picture of her lying on Brenda's pale chest: she doesn't have a blueberry muffin rash or a small head or need oxygen. I know I shouldn't feel relieved about her typicality—that one of our culture's most damaging lies is that "normal" doesn't inherently include the atypical. But still, it's true: I feel relief. And I realize it's relief that Michael and Brenda won't be facing CMV's unknowns—and the personal impact of its not being known.

Because it's not the symptoms of CMV in Anna that have shredded my nerves most. It's that no one knows. Which feels to me like no one cares.

I hear someone calling me.

"Ma'am? Did it work?" It's the Verizon lady, whom I'd entirely forgotten.

When I answer her, I'm crying. "It worked! My phone works! My brother had a baby! I'm looking at her now, and she's beautiful. They're going to call her Addie."

"Well, this is definitely going to be the highlight of my day," the lady says.

I'm laughing and crying, and I tell her, "Mine, too."

3

Two days after my niece is born, it's Anna's first birthday. Which means it's time to go to the hospital for her well check. I'm excited to show Dr. Vastola and the older nurse I swim laps with, Kim, how well Anna is doing. As I pull into the parking lot, narrating that we're *driving-driving-slowing-stopping,* I also realize what the tone of my own voice is telling me: that even if the news of Zika is weighing me down, I'm still way stabler than I was last summer. Zaley is with me, too, and though she's now sat through over one hundred appointments for Anna, she's still excited to come along. She loves nurses, doctors, and therapists, and she absorbs, verbatim, most of the things they say.

Inside, we go to the receptionist's window, where I tell the employee, wincing inside, that yes, we are still self-pay. (A fisherman has to buy his insurance, and there's no policy we can purchase that will allow in-network coverage of Anna's doctors in both Colorado and Alaska.) I can already feel the stress of opening envelopes from this place, the line items unnamed and unexplained, all the phone calls I'll have to make, wondering how it's possible that we live in a country with so much money and so many healthcare companies and so little consideration of our sanity as the very foundation of our health. But we have no choice—we take the elevator up to the second floor and enter an exam room to wait.

How many times have I sat with Anna in these rooms, stripped her to her diaper, looked lovingly at her tiny, puffing belly, her expectant eyes, her air-handling hands? How much she has uncurled since last summer—her breasts have flattened out, her wrists even have a slight marshmallowy softness if you poke one with your finger. She's wearing a red headband, and now she can sign *milk, Zaley, chicken,* and *all done.*

When Dr. Vastola walks in, he's taken aback. He can see Anna's still small, but she is sitting, smiling, aware, and thriving. "Wow, she looks really great," he says, and Zaley, who is nodding and looking at Anna, says, "Doesn't she?"—so accustomed to this exchange, she can be me, by proxy.

Dr. Vastola isn't alone. A medical student with a hip haircut— longer on one side than the other—introduces herself as Kate and stands next to Dr. Vastola to observe. She's in her sixth year of an M.D./Ph.D. program at the University of Washington—the number- one med school in the country for primary care—and when I tell her Anna has congenital CMV, she looks at me, unfamiliar with the term.

"I've never heard of it," she says.

Dr. Vastola looks at me, and I look at him. "Well," I begin, and the numbers and stats are coming fast, before Kate stops me and says, "Can you hang on just one second? I want to go get a notebook and a pen."

When Kate returns, Dr. Vastola begins his exam. He acknowledges that I'm right—Anna doesn't have any sign of teeth—but he also sees how reactive she is to sound, to his voice, to the light he dances in her eyes. Then he does the trick where he ignites Zaley's index finger with the ophthalmoscope shining behind it, and when he has her blow it out with her breath, Anna snaps her head toward it and laughs and laughs. Next, he puts his stethoscope into Zaley's ears and glides the diaphragm over Anna's chest. A minute later Zaley's eyes beam bright with recognition: this is the sound of her sister's beating heart.

While I believe most doctors work *from* a place of goodness, Dr. Vastola also works *toward* it. He gathers details about our family from Zaley, inquiring about our lives outside the room: what does she like to do on the airplane, does she enjoy fishing, which of Anna's therapies does Zaley like going to best? He never seems goofy or impatient, just genuinely interested. As he shows Zaley every tool he has, I pick up where I left off, explaining to Kate, who's now sitting down, the lack of knowledge about CMV during pregnancy, the noncommittal stance of ACOG, the critical timing of early identification so that babies with symptoms can receive treatment. When Dr. Vastola has gotten all of Zaley's answers and Anna's vitals, he leans over to Kate and says, "This is not your typical one-year appointment with a mom."

Damn right it's not. And I can tell Dr. Vastola is complimenting me, not suggesting that I'm overbearing or wrong. He's saying to Kate that I'm the expert in the room. And that's when I realize I'm doing something I've not done before: I'm educating medical professionals, in detail, about congenital CMV. While nine months ago, I barely knew how to talk to my neighbors, by now, these facts have been burned into my brain. And with my research has come a confidence and a certainty that it's information everyone should have.

I also know now that there's no difference between a mother's brain and her doctor's—they are both coiled, complex machines that grasp and sort information, that accrue numbers and experiences, that hypothesize and draw conclusions, though often, in Western medicine, the doctor-patient relationship seems to place parental knowledge—especially a mother's—on a rung below the professional's. One primary care physician whose writing I love, Dr. Suzanne Koven, explains that "the hidden curriculum" of medical school is "the teaching that our patients are somehow fundamentally different from us and we from them." In her excellent book, *Letter to a Young Female Physician,* she insists that this assumption should be dismantled and dropped.

Dr. Vastola seems to understand what Dr. Suzanne Koven does: that the people they serve are walking around with the same highly functioning brains and quietly broken hearts as theirs. Kate looks like she knows this, too, and I will be forever grateful to her for being the first—and one of the only—medical professionals who openly, actively showed me that she was willing to learn more. And that she could learn it from me.

Because as a mother, I have never felt like an expert at anything, until now, with Kate sitting humbly in a plastic chair, her eyes at the same level as mine.

While it's true that doctors devote huge chunks of their lives to school and residency, rotations and clinicals, and they see more patients and symptoms in a day than a lay person does in a year, we, as parents, have something else going for us that our kids' medical practitioners don't: immersion. We are immersed not only in our children but in the medical topics that concern them.

When a doctor goes on their lunch break, they talk with colleagues and spouses; they read journals in their specialty (which is very rarely CMV). When a CMV mom gets a lunch break (hah—I joke!), we're showing our kids how to properly swallow liquid through a honey-bear bottle, reading a CMV study with one eye while watching our toddler with the other, and wondering what specialist we've failed to include in our child's mostly parent-directed care. We aren't practitioners because we aren't *practicing;* we are *living*—with our lives as the clinic, and no break from our patient.

We, the parents of children with CMV, also live through the symptoms of its dismissal. We remember the provider who sighs ever so slightly when leaving the room; we notice the quickening pace of an appointment, after the letters CMV leave our lips. We have to answer when a health professional asks something like *So is she okay?* wondering by what metrics they expect us to quantify our child's okay-ness: Are they asking if she's not disabled? Are they asking if she's not blind, not deaf, not delayed? We are catalogs of these lapses, choosing to be defeated or impelled by them, depending on the day.

Once in the winter, I'd had the unfortunate experience of needing to address two medical mistakes. I'd taken Anna to the pediatrician's office for a bad cold, and the doctor had called an ambulance after we arrived because Anna was dangerously low on oxygen, her skin going a sickly gray. When the paramedics arrived, they took Anna from me and placed her facing backward in her car seat inside the ambulance, where neither the paramedic nor I could see her face. It was snowy and rush hour, so we couldn't get to the hospital fast, and their equipment couldn't consistently register an infant's pulse. Every minute or so, a long beeping filled the ambulance, as though Anna had flatlined and died.

"I'd rather ride where I can see her," I said, unbuckling, but the paramedic put up his hand.

"I can see her *fontelle* from where I'm sitting," he said. He meant her soft spot, which was barely visible under the canopy of her car seat, and he proceeded to tell me what I already knew: that you can see the pulse of an infant where the skin over the soft spot rises and falls.

"I know," I said. "It's called a font-*a*-nelle."

"No," he retorted. "It's called a *fontelle*."

We rode the rest of the way in silence, with me sitting on the floor in front of my child.

At the ER, over the sound of the suctioning tool that vacuumed the mucus painfully out of Anna's lungs, the admitting doctor said Anna would need to be catheterized to check her for an infection, and I told him she had CMV. Then he asked if I'd contracted CMV from *kitty litter* during pregnancy.

"No," I told him. "CMV comes from toddlers, not cats. And unlike toxoplasmosis, which affects about one in ten thousand newborns, CMV infects one in two hundred babies in the U.S."

He excused himself, and I asked the nurse not to send him back. Instead, I texted Cole, Luke's brother, who happened to be a urology resident at the same hospital at the time. When Cole showed up, in a suit and a tie, he leaned against the counter, as if he had a long time to spend, not patients and paperwork waiting upstairs. He called another urologist on the phone, in front of me, requesting that an expert catheterize Anna because she was still so small.

Of course, Anna was his niece, but he made the conscious choice to treat Anna like his own—a simple tweak that could drastically reform the field of medicine. All night, I held Anna while she was hot and quivering in the hospital bed, while my friend Mia, on her birthday, drove through the mounting snow to keep me company. She pulled little camping tins of chocolates and nuts out of her diaper bag to get us through the lonely hours when the hospital cafeteria wasn't open for midnight snacks. While doctors around us performed surgeries, reset bones, and saved lives, we mothers did the other important work: we watched the green lines drawn by Anna's heart on the screen, repositioned the tubes in her nose, and never left the room.

Anna's life happens in the cocoon of mine. Her disease first knew me intimately, entered through me as its host. And the best doctors understand me as her chrysalis—I am protective, prone to tearing, and a necessity to her transformation.

———

"I could go on and on," I tell Kate, the medical student, in Sitka. "But I'm sure you have other patients to see."

Kate's eyes are unblinking, her pen is poised above a small paper pad. She sets them in her lap, draws in a deep breath, and says, "I just can't believe I didn't know about this."

She admits she knew about cytomegalovirus from the TORCH acronym for infectious diseases that some women are tested for during pregnancy, when they have markers of infection. TORCH stands for toxoplasmosis, other viruses (like syphilis or varicella), rubella, cytomegalovirus, and herpes. But I won't learn till later that often, in medical school, these diseases aren't parsed out from each other and studied in-depth, individually. Or that doctors rarely even order the TORCH test because it's so limited in its usefulness and usually requires much more specific follow-up testing. Kate says she definitely never heard about CMV's volatility during pregnancy nor that it transmits through toddlers.

"Do you think you'd be comfortable giving me your email address?" she asks me, "so I can ask you some questions later?"

"Ask me more questions?" I question her back, smiling. I have never heard a healthcare provider pose this request. "For sure! Yes!"

When we leave, I can hear Dr. Vastola still talking to Kate. He's not watering down the issue of CMV or stating how many kids with it end up unaffected. I can hear him say, "CMV is a very serious disease." This is the crux of it: simple, direct, and yet so very contested among doctors who know less.

———

When Luke gets home that evening, I ask him if I can run to the library. And there, with a newfound sense of authority, I write. I write about waking up to the hollow croaks of the ravens on our roof.

I write about the vowels of Anna's voice in the morning, calling to me in tones she cannot hear. I write about my constant navigation between sound and silence. Not only does the writing of it bring me pleasure, it's also the beginning of a piece that will lead to opportunities I never could have imagined.

4

To teach a deaf child to speak, the first step is introducing the Ling sounds—six sounds that span all the frequencies of speech. To do so, I hold up an object, then plop the object into a bucket after I've made its respective noise. There's an Alaska Airlines toy plane that says "aah"; a gray rubber mouse says "eee"; a plastic ice cream cone says "mmm"; a ghost says "ooh"; a snake goes "sss"; and a tiny baby doll says "shhh" under the blanket of a Kleenex. The idea is to condition Anna: eventually, she will make the sound of each object before dropping it into a container. Zaley helps with this game, and our new AVT, Joanna, facilitates the process now that Nancy has retired.

We meet with Joanna on Zoom before the rest of the world knows what Zoom is. Sometimes I rig the iPad inside a spiraled, metallic lamp base to free my hands, where it delivers us to Joanna at such a slant that I catch Joanna tilting her head. Sometimes Zaley is so interested in showing Joanna an object of zero significance (a wooden spoon! a quarter!), she blocks the webcam with the object entirely until I can lift her away. Sometimes I hate the option of remote therapy, even though I love the therapists who suffer through this distance and chaos to serve Anna's needs.

We've also started doing in-person OT with a woman named Tori who has cute clothes and two young kids of her own and I just plain love her. Tori brings foam balance beams for Anna and doctor kits for Zaley, and she never refuses a cup of coffee. She rolls Anna's feet over a soup can to stimulate them so they'll come unclawed. She massages each of Anna's toes, while Anna melts with contentment in her lap.

But no one can tell me what I most want to know, which is if one day Anna will spread out those toes and walk.

I know enough about disability narratives—from the ones I've read and the ones I've witnessed in the Deaf community and from having an uncle, my dad's brother Don, who became a paraplegic after being shot and never regained the use of his legs—that I shouldn't arrange our lives around Anna being able to "overcome." That some bodies don't do what other bodies do ever. That to expect this is to perpetuate the prejudice that people aren't whole unless they live in a standardized body instead of their own.

But as much as I want to honor Anna's unique experience, it would also be dishonest to say that I didn't care about her mobility. I want her to be mobile, in her own way, on her own time, whenever that might be.

At thirteen months, Anna is just starting her own version of crawling, which Zaley and I find intolerably cute. She pulls herself forward with two hands, one in a fist, and bicycles her legs behind her, till one of her feet sticks. Then, she worms her way toward the object we have planted a few feet in front of her—usually a hot pink ball that lights up blue. Mostly Anna just likes to sit. This isn't a passive act. She sits in the middle of the room with her legs sticking straight out from her hips. She sits under where Zaley is in action, mixing food coloring and water into four margarita cups, stirring them around with a serious look, then leaning down to offer Anna careful sips.

Partly to serve Anna's needs but also to remind myself that I can't rush Anna toward anything, I've found one additional therapist in Sitka who practices the Feldenkrais method. (Moshe Feldenkrais was the physicist who actually taught Anat Baniel all about neuroplasticity in the brain). This local therapist, named Martina, has an unrelated day job; she just does this on the side.

I can tell by the way Martina moves Anna, so gently I want to go to sleep, that she isn't here for the money (which she often refuses, and we pay her in salmon instead). She doesn't have any kids, and when she's sitting with Anna between her knees, I tell her I stay home with mine.

Instead of extending pity or asking what else I do, Martina says, "Thank you."

And I say, "For what?"

And she says, "For contributing a great thing to society."

———

Sometimes the most life-changing things are simple sentences the person speaking them barely even remembers.

For days, I think about what Martina said: *Thank you for contributing a great thing to society.*

I'm deeply moved that she sees motherhood as that thing. And I don't believe any mother needs to do anything else to feel she's contributing something of great import to the world. But when I think about her words over the course of the next few weeks, I'm also thinking about something else.

Ever since I was in third grade, I wanted to be a writer. My third-grade teacher was a severe and dedicated instructor named Donna Weber, who had short swoops of brown-gray hair and long black nostrils, and who put a noticeable emphasis on "the language arts"— the very phrase whetting my imagination and my sense of purpose. We read silently under our desks, we read to each other in pairs, we wrote stories for homework, and then we read them aloud in front of the class. But I could never write enough. It's all I wanted to do. I wrote one story that was twenty-four pages long on loose-leaf, stapled it proudly way too many times along its edge, then turned it in for Mrs. Weber to read. I don't remember what she said about the story, but I remember that it only felt complete because I'd turned it in to her.

I didn't want it back, I told her, and so she kept it. I loved this; I felt like a writer for the first time, because I had an audience, a person to whom I could contribute what I'd made.

———

There isn't a word in English for this compulsion to give something freely, to desire to contribute something of import to another person or society. But there is in Hebrew, and it's a word associated with my grandma's name, Ruth—which is Anna's middle name, too.

In the Old Testament, Ruth was a Moabite woman who lost all the male members of her family, including her husband. She could

have left town and remarried someone somewhere else, as would
have been expected at the time, but instead she devoted herself to
her mother-in-law, Naomi, with remarkably loyalty and sacrifice.
She told Naomi—who suggested fervently that Ruth leave—that no
matter what, she would remain by her side.

The Hebrew word for the quality Ruth exuded is *hesed*—which
means more than just loving-kindness or honor or generosity. *Hesed*
means a sense of love so great you *act*. And you act on behalf of
someone else in need. *Hesed* comes from a deeper place than social
expectations or responsibilities. *Hesed* is the call and the response, the
way of being and its delivery.

Everyone is capable of *hesed,* but far too few people know
what it is. I think if people knew they had a penchant for *hesed,*
they would approach every opportunity—parenthood, creativity,
medicine—differently.

As a child, I knew I could write, but I could not put words to my
desire to do it—I wouldn't know about *hesed* for another thirty years,
when we named Anna what we did. I only knew, after my third-
grade teacher gave me the gift of my first acceptance, that writing
was what I wanted to do forever. That it could be both self-fulfilling
and self-giving was something I could sense.

It wasn't until my senior year of college at Tulane University,
in New Orleans, that I got to take my first class in creative writing. The teacher was a poet named Peter Cooley, who came in late
and disheveled on the first day of class, rubbing his upright grayish
hair with the heel of one hand. He was short, with big wild eyes
behind thick square glasses. We read mostly poems and short stories
he pulled out from a bursting briefcase, but he never had us read
his own words—writing that revealed how tender, how full of pain
and love he truly was. He brought in guest writers, now published,
whom he had taught. When they talked about their own work, he
leaned back in his chair, his eyes ablaze with admiration. I wanted
to be them.

At the end of the semester, when I went to visit him during his
office hours, I was shocked by the cinematic mess of his space—like

some half-mad professor holed up in a tree, he'd spread manuscripts all over the floor, stacked books literally from floor to ceiling. A single window was nearly crowded out by towers of literature. I loved it. I told him I was already enrolled in the English literature master's program that would start the following fall, but that I had made a mistake. I wanted to pursue creative writing. I wanted to be a writer instead.

"Maybe you should drop out," he said, bending down and rustling under his desk.

"What?" I asked.

"Drop out of the master's program," he said. "Maybe look into an MFA instead."

So I did exactly what he said: I dropped out of the master's program that very day. I applied to master of fine arts programs—three-year graduate programs somewhere between a master's degree and a Ph.D., where you usually produce a book. But then, a few months later, Hurricane Katrina hit, and I decided I couldn't leave. I ended up teaching high school English and creative writing in the bayou, an hour away. I loved those kids, and I loved introducing them to published writers who were dreamers like them.

Two years later, though, I knew in my heart that I needed to leave the heat and the dysfunction of my relationships in the South. I applied to a different MFA program, a program in Alaska, which sounded dreamily cold. Then I met Luke in that church, on a short trip home from New Orleans, and I couldn't believe his stability, what he did for a living, and where.

In my MFA program, I did write a book. It was about loving a place and needing to leave it. But when I pitched it, in a bookstore in Denver, to a literary agent visiting from New York, he had zero interest in my story. After supposedly reading my manuscript, he made no mention of it; instead, he wanted to tell me about one crazy night he'd had on Bourbon Street during a bachelor party. When I shook his hand to leave, I intended to conceal my woundedness and exit as gracefully as I could. I ended up falling backward over my chair.

So despite that book I'd already written, despite the falling down, I do still want to be a writer—and now, more than ever, because of congenital CMV. But in the writing world, rejection is, by my rough calculations, about 99 percent more common than acceptance. And I'm not sure I have it in me to pitch a book whose central subject, CMV, is already so overtly rejected and also so very close to my heart.

Then one night I look up Dr. Cooley's work again to find my favorite poem of his, "The One Certain Thing," which starts with the line "A day will come I'll watch you reading this."

And then I know: literature is an act of *hesed,* one that can reach us at our lowest, hoist us up, drastically reroute our lives. And I know I will write this down: the research, the rage, the silences, the sorrow. And maybe one day, the remedies.

I do get asked to write something. But it isn't for a publication. It's for Kate, the med student at SEARHC. As a visiting medical student, she'll be giving a presentation at the end of her rotation in a few weeks. And she wants to give the presentation on congenital CMV.

She wants studies, and I'm sure I send too many. She wants our story, and I try to rein it in. She wants a picture of Anna and Zaley, and when I explain to Zaley what I'm working on, she picks out ten photographs for Kate, then proceeds to imitate Kate for the next few weeks.

When the day of the presentation arrives, though, it doesn't happen. Kate emails me: *Dr. Vastola has delayed it,* she writes, and my heart descends. But then I read why: he has postponed it out of concern that not enough doctors could attend.

A week later I get an email from Kate. I tell Zaley I need her to be quiet while I read it—which she is not—but I open the email anyway. Kate has given her presentation, and it went great.

All the docs were really interested, she writes. *They were shocked with the stats on prevalence and lack of knowledge among women. And our OB-GYN said he's hoping ACOG comes around on the issue*—a statement I can hardly believe.

I'm beaming when I close my computer and finally turn my attention to Zaley, who is standing with her arms at her sides, her hands inside the too-long sleeves of my white fleece coat. Her hair is parted way down on the side of her head and swooped sideways in a dramatic comb-over, appearing as though it's cut asymmetrically. I realize instantly who she's pretending to be.

"My name is Kate, and I'm an M-D-P-H-D," Zaley says, just right. "What can you tell me about congenital CMV?"

5

Luke wants to go on a hike. Usually, on his days off, we like to have coffee on the deck (or under the tarp) while the girls point at the big planes taking off from the runway and the small ones landing on the sea. But Derek and Jules and their kids are going hiking on Kruzof Island, where the dormant volcano sits, squat and flat-topped and bear-infested across the sound. Luke doesn't say how many miles this hike will entail, but the destination is a place I've wanted to go for years—a hard-to-access beach with white sand surrounded by old-growth forests called Sealion Cove.

I love to hike, and we rarely do it anymore. But I'm hesitant to go. I'm anxious about the details: When will the girls nap? What food can I bring that Anna will eat? What if it rains and it sucks and I miss the opportunity to write or go for a swim? I want to be adventurous, but something about parenting feels so inversely related to it. I can tell this is a problem with parenting itself, not with my children. I watch Zaley, who's naked and sprinting back and forth down the hallway, shouting, "Beach day! Beach day!" and I know I could have her sense of freedom if I could shake off my anxiety. I'm not even afraid of danger; I'm afraid that if I don't look like I'm in control—if my children don't behave, or if they don't nap, or if they're an utter mess the next day—then I, and my children, are failures.

Luke, on the other hand, has no such illusions. He expects failure, actually relishes it as opportunity. Once in the spring, I'd forgotten to dress Zaley in her jammies for pajama day at school. Upon drop-off, when I saw all the other preschoolers in their comfy sleepers and Zaley in her stiff uniform, I was so disappointed—so in fear of Zaley's disappointment—that I rushed right home to grab her pajamas and bring them back to her at school.

"You know, you don't need to do that," Luke had said, when I got home and told him why I was blasting out the door with Zaley's PJs in my hand. "She'll actually be better off if you don't."

Then he told me about his first day of high school: it was a ropes course day, and at his Catholic high school, the students were allowed the rare privilege of wearing T-shirts, tennis shoes, and shorts. But Luke, having missed the memo, showed up in formal attire—dress pants, an oxford shirt, a blazer, and a tie.

Luke's mom wouldn't have entertained the thought of rescuing him. She had four younger kids to take to various schools. Anita knew that Luke would grow in character if left to solve his own problems. And that navigating his own way through them would lend him a lack of entitlement to some altogether assembled life. So that day, his first day of high school, Luke wore his dress clothes all day long and climbed the ropes in his starched shirt and pants.

Maybe because of that embarrassing day, he would end up becoming student body president of his high school, and later he'd win a full-ride leadership scholarship to a prestigious university—a scholarship he just barely redeemed, because he was fishing in Alaska till the day before college started, when his dad told him he'd better get his ass back.

What Luke knew was that what looks like failure can actually be good parenting. That a family who looks perfect is probably working way too hard to maintain that illusion.

So when Luke says we should go to Sealion Cove, I try to channel his disregard for trivial details, his distaste for the attempt to control. Emma and Johnny will entertain Zaley on the hike, he says, and he'll carry her when she pouts. He'll pack a bunch of food, and Anna will nap in the Ergo on one of our backs. Also, Max will come along.

Max is Luke's youngest brother—the one who had no soft spot at birth, then surgery, then seizures for many years after—and a few weeks ago, he flew up to deckhand for Luke. Max drives the *Drifter* when Luke's too tired, he filets all the fish on a white stand at the back of the boat, and in general, he stands next to Luke all day, chatting about elk hunting, the girl he likes, his grades, his life plans—which, for now, are to come up here like Luke and fish.

Max is seventeen. He's huge-smiled and handsome and charming (so much so, the following May a girl in Sitka will fly him up to attend her prom), and in the evenings, rather than retreating to his bedroom to text friends at home, he plays his guitar on the couch, wrestles with Zaley on the living room floor, or swims with her in the hot tub while I start dinner. Max imparts a levity to parenting that feels harder, I think, in the absence of extended family.

So I pack light and throw naps to the wind. We meet at the harbor, where Jules looks like she's packed for a week.

———

I know our life would be easier without Sitka in it. But it would also be more typical, less beautiful. In the same way that I wouldn't trade Anna for anything, I fear replacing Sitka with a life where we'd be more ordinary.

Jules and Derek are a good study for me. They've made the same seasonal dynamic as ours work for close to thirty years, and their children look forward to fishing season all year long to escape the heat and frenetic pace of life down south. Johnny and Emma love Sitka. They can catch the biggest fish their friends back home have ever seen. They can do puzzles or read books or play pickup basketball at the Hames Center all day and have nowhere to be. They don't have obligatory sports practices, long car rides, or a lawn full of pointless grass to mow. They can drive up Harbor Mountain and see the world from up there.

"Don't you miss summer back home, where it's warm?" I ask Emma, on the way to Sealion Cove.

"NO WAY!" she says. At twelve, Emma is taller than me and also more optimistic, less weather-obsessed, more Alaskan.

I find it deeply comforting that she never feels she's missing out. I want us to be a family like theirs—and in some ways we are. But I can't tell if I love our lives less than other people do up here.

"It's because your kids are so young," Jules always says. And she's probably right. But how can I know if I'll feel this way in ten years unless we spend the next ten years doing the same difficult thing?

———

I had imagined that the boat ride to Kruzof, so visible in the distance from the parking lot at Sea Mart, would be about ten minutes long. In actuality, it's about an hour and a half. We are aiming for Kalinin Bay, where we'll anchor the boat in deep water, then pile into a small Zodiac raft to be transported, by groups of two or three, to the trailhead for the hike. From the back of Derek's boat, where I'm nursing Anna and Luke is asking Zaley not to jump up and down on the bench or she'll hit her head, I hear Jules say something to Derek about the hike being 2.5 miles, one way.

"Did I just hear you say this hike is five miles round trip?" I ask.

"Not quite," says Derek, turning around and grinning, which means it's probably even longer than that.

Jules doesn't say much the rest of the ride because she's busy with something else. She's reading something I printed before we left the house: it's a long essay I've been working on that begins with Anna's birth and suggests that Zika is a decoy blocking our view of CMV in the United States. I've interviewed Dr. Gail Demmler-Harrison over the phone for the piece.

The kids are on the bow of the boat in the wind, reenacting the wide-armed scene from *The Titanic,* when Jules swivels around in a captain's chair next to Derek. Her mouth is taut. There's a fire in her eyes. "Megs," she says. "The leading cause of birth defects, and no one knows about it? Benevolent deception is bullshit. Someone will publish this. They have to."

―――――

The Zodiac is small and tippy, and I didn't bring Anna's waterproof implants. I'm holding her as steady as I can as we approach car-size gray rocks that jut out of the Pacific in dramatic slants. Zaley is on the rocks already, having taken the first raft trip with Max and Johnny and Emma, and they are jumping from one rock to the next, sliding down the smooth faces of stone beside water so deep that if Zaley fell in, I would never see her again.

I try not to watch. I try not to say anything to Luke to indicate that if I had known we'd be two hours in and not yet on land, I probably would have stayed home. Five minutes later the Zodiac hits stone, and Luke helps me down. Beyond the rocks, pale grass gleams in a meadow, shifting into lines and then straightening itself in the wind. Berries line either side of a skinny dirt trail. And as soon as we start walking, I see that the kids aren't the only ones interested in picking them: a football field length to our left, four brown bears are walking idly through hedges of their own, toothing the branches and pulling off the fruit.

I have imagined this moment before, the flood of fear I would feel, the instinct to run. But in my head, there was never another mother with me. Sometimes I think that if I always had another mom by my side, my own mom or a friend, it would be so much better than it is. It is Jules who turns my fear to ease, Jules who is tall and confident and never afraid of bears, who gives a quick, bellowing "Hey bear!" before they look up at us, unimpressed, as we vanish between the trees.

———

The trails in Sitka are maintained by million-dollar grants awarded to a nonprofit called Sitka Trail Works. Where you might expect wilderness hikes to be all bushwhacking and misery, the trails around Sitka are often beautifully designed with miles-long boardwalks that ascend craggy mountains and cross boggy valleys. The Sealion Cove hike is no exception—some of it is unmaintained and slick with mud, but other stretches are equipped with the pleasant side-by-side two-by-sixes so common to hiking around here. When the terrain gets steeper, the boards rise up in a step, or two, or ten, and sometimes a felled tree is cut into a staircase with the bottom side kept flat and the top side notched out into steps.

The kids lead the way. We pass big bear prints and a lake, winding through dense, unfamiliar terrain. While I listen to the happy knock-knock noises our Xtratufs make on the wood, I realize Zaley is nowhere near me, bounding ahead with the older kids and out of sight. And because I can't see her, I'm not trying to gauge the safety of her every move. Watching her appear smaller ahead, I realize that somewhere along the line, I've confused protecting her with controlling her.

Glancing down at Anna in the pack under my chin, I know that if I'd understood this during pregnancy—that protection is love, but believing we can control any outcome of our children is not—CMV would have been just one more species to understand in the brimming wilderness of parenting.

Even though Zaley is typically hesitant in new situations, clinging to me in any kind of foreign territory, she must sense a change in me while we're hiking. Because on this walk, she never stops. When we reach the muskeg—a soggy meadow where the mossy ground literally bounces under your feet—she's like a fairy dancing in the woods. Here there are carpets of blueberries; short, stunted pine trees that corkscrew up from the spongy ground; and grandfather's beard that looks like Spanish moss in New Orleans, hanging down pastel green and wispy from the branches of trees. Soon under a stand of hemlocks, the space beneath the trunks seems to suggest we're about to reach an opening—and then there it is: at the edge of the trees is the most expansive beach I have ever seen.

It appears as if in a black and white movie: the sand is such a white, it looks like it's made of confectioners' sugar, not something that once was shells and stone. The water, frequented by friends of ours who are surfers, rushes toward us in long white chutes that crash open on the pewter shore. There are no people but us, and the view is so stunning and we are all so tired that we all just sit down—some on a twenty-foot piece of driftwood, made holey by birds and time, and some of us directly on the sand.

It has taken us about five hours to get to this place, from door to water. I look at Luke, and I crunch my eyebrows at him because this is my way of acknowledging that he could say right now, *I told you this would be worth it,* which he never does.

While Zaley and Luke comb the shore for treasures, I sit back watching them, wondering who taught me that white-knuckling every minute might make me look like a good mother to well-rested, well-behaved kids. It certainly wasn't my mom. When I was a kid, we played outside all the time without her, ate noodles every day, watched TV without her knowing how many minutes we'd watched. Maybe I've been so awash in the anxiety of our parenting culture, so governed by worthless competition and impossible perfectionism, that I've forgotten—or I never knew in the first place—that my capability and my capacity have nothing to do with the way

I look, the way my kids behave, the diseases they have, or the way a day begins to deteriorate.

Pleasure, I see in the whitewashed beauty of Sealion Cove, comes not from flawlessly behaved kids or a job well done but from seeing all that we've become. Luke is walking toward me on the beach, Zaley is trotting next to him, and Anna is in his arms. All of a sudden, Zaley stops and picks something up. She holds it up. It's a heart-shaped rock. And now she's running back to me crying because she has sand inside her socks. What a perfect metaphor for how I feel about Alaska.

It's like my friend from Italy once said: "I loved becoming a mom because it meant I was bigger than myself."

Before we leave Sealion Cove, we eat a quick lunch of smoked salmon and crackers and take one last look at the minty green tunnels made by the cresting waves. Then we start the long march back to the boat. Zaley sleeps in a hiking backpack on Luke's back the whole three hours. Anna watches the clouds, my mouth, the start and stop of trees. I do get stung, twice, by bees, but we don't get eaten, we don't get back to the dock too late. Max puts Zaley on his shoulders, and we trudge up the steep blue boat ramp, ready for hot showers and home.

When the girls are in bed that night, I make my final changes to the essay Jules encouraged me to submit. Then I open my email server. I type the address for the *New York Times* opinion editor, I attach my essay, and I hit send.

After I've sent out a piece of writing, the waiting period has a sweetness to it, when my hope is at its highest. Which is not so different from the time before Anna does any new thing.

I'm enjoying this in-between time when one day, before it's time to go home, I hear it:

"Mom."

I'm standing in the kitchen.

Not believing who might have said it, I come around to the other side of the island. There's just Anna in the entryway, her arms prop-ping her up on a package of toilet paper. "What?" I say.

"Mom." Anna says, looking straight at me, like she's been saying it all along.

"Zaley!" I scream. "Come here!"

I hear some shuffling back in Zaley's bedroom, and then her running feet. She's wearing a fly-fishing vest that goes down to her knees.

"Anna, baby," I say, kneeling down on the floor. "Can you say it again?"

Anna plops down. Now her hands are free, her fingers are spread, and she raises her thumb to her chin. She signs it to me—*Mom*—and then, she says it again: "MOM."

Zaley and I are giggling now, nearly hysterical, googly-eyed with shock. She rolls over me, steamroller style, unable to contain her excitement, then rolls all the way down the hallway, then back again.

Anna is quiet now. Her mouth is closed, her eyes are bright, her legs are two parallel, straight lines. She's smiling her sneaky smile, well aware, it seems, of her silence. And her voice.

6

Once we're back home in Colorado, Anna has what's called a "language burst." She says "ot-ot-ot" when she taps my coffee cup with her palm, then withdraws her hand with an open mouth. She shrieks "Dada!" as soon as she spots Luke. She also says "chicken" now when she signs it (thumb and index finger pecking, beaklike, at the hand). When Zaley bursts in the door from prekindergarten every day at noon, Anna yells out "Ay-zee!" for her name.

I do not, however, feel the same progress in my own land of words. I've been checking my email obsessively for the last few months, waiting for a response from *The New York Times,* and no response has come. In October, though, I go to their homepage, and my vision goes dizzy for a moment when the letters *CMV* catch my eyes.

There's an article before me titled "CMV Is a Greater Threat to Infants Than Zika but Far Less Often Discussed." When I click the article with shaky fingers, there's a picture of a CMV mom with her daughter, and a quick glance down from there, I see that one of the providers who's been interviewed for the piece is Dr. Gail Demmler-Harrison in Texas.

I want to feel gratitude that a writer is paying attention to CMV. But I want to cry that the story wasn't written by me. Did this journalist get wind of my piece on CMV, then track down the story for herself? Or were the timing and content a coincidence, set into motion by Zika, over the summer? I know I won't know. I swallow my pain and my pride and scroll back up. I linger on the first picture—a photo of a CMV mom named Erica and her child, Evelyn, who's in a wheelchair and being lifted into a school bus. The CMV story is not mine alone to tell, I remind myself. If anything, it belongs more to these families whose children are bearing most of its weight. So I sit up straight. And I read.

I start at the byline. The author is named Catherine Saint Louis, and she's a staff writer at *The New York Times*. She deftly explains the complexities of CMV and its lack of recognition. She shares the opinions of four mothers in the piece, and the stories of their girls who span the spectrum of CMV's symptoms: Evelyn is deaf and completely disabled; Jane and Daisy are deaf without other manifestations; and Kaitlyn is like Anna, deaf with moderate delays.

It's when I get to the part about ACOG that the blood floods back up to my brain. In the article, Dr. Christopher Zahn, the vice president for practice at ACOG, is quoted saying the two things I always hear in opposition to being honest about CMV: one, that universal precautions haven't proven effective enough to prevent the disease. "Come on!" I say aloud, to no one. "CMV is a *virus*!" I know that scientific research has proven handwashing to be extremely effective. I also know what Dr. Karen Fowler, an epidemiologist in Alabama, told me once over the phone: "You have to understand the love/hate relationship the medical field has with behavioral interventions. They don't believe in them as a whole. It's hard to change human behavior which is correct; they'd rather have a medical solution—a drug or a vaccine." And finally, I know the unspoken reason universal precautions haven't been "proven" to prevent CMV, as Dr. Zahn suggests: CMV studies have never been awarded enough funding—therefore enough participants—for the FDA to deem them sufficient.

The second thing he says in the article is just a rewording of irresponsibility: "There are so many topics to cover during pregnancy, that this is often driven by what patients are most worried about." I hate this deferral, which seems cowardly and blaming. What Dr. Zahn is saying is that OBs cover what the morning news tells us to fear, not what is statistically and scientifically much more likely to be disabling. And because the piece is written as a news piece, not an opinion piece, I hate that his comments might register objectively— and worse, as unobjectionable.

While the rest of the article does make a case for the effectiveness of counseling women about CMV, I realize that the real story—the exposé of medical paternalism; the impact of medical silence on our children; the impassioned argument—is not going to be adequately voiced unless it's voiced by someone personally experiencing it.

Looking it up, I find that even though Catherine Saint Louis successfully published her story about a maternal-fetal disease in *The New York Times,* she did so amidst a serious gender disparity: of the journalists at *The New York Times* with annual salaries of $150,000 or more, only 36 percent are women. And, I read on, this is a trend that infects the entire news industry: of all newswire articles published by the Associated Press and Reuters, women are the authors of only 31 percent of them. Even if you take writers out of the equation and look instead at what the public reads, the same neglect of women's issues is true: women are the subjects of only 24 percent of global news pieces.

How does a mother like me, never on staff anywhere, with two small children at my feet, bring attention to an invisible disease that begins silently, in the dark, invisible orb of the uterus?

I have only one connection at my fingertips, so I use it: I email Catherine Saint Louis, the writer of the piece in the *Times*. I tell her about Anna, about my pitch to her publication, about the story I still have to tell.

To my great surprise, she emails right back. She provides me with the name and email of another editor there who may consider a personal essay about CMV. When I look up the guidelines for submitting to this other department—the health column, called "Well"—I see that I'll need to cut my essay by about 90 percent. Always one to overdo things, I know this will take me longer than it did to write the original. But I will. Because this is what we do: we shorten the CMV story for the parents of other preschoolers who are on their way home for lunch, for our children's doctors who are on their way to see their next patient.

In the meantime, I pitch a similar article to *The Denver Post,* where I was once a regularly contributing freelance columnist. My editor, Barbara, can't believe the story about CMV and says yes—I should start writing the piece. But my heart sinks when, about halfway into drafting the article, I get an email from Barbara. The managing editor above her is not comfortable with me writing the story. *You're too close to it,* Barbara relays.

I email her back, a plea:

> *Some of the facts in the story took me months to find—I dug for days through articles in a small library in Alaska, while paying for a babysitter, to write a story I will get paid nothing to write. It isn't about money of course, it's about this being my story, my child— even if it's not traditionally the mother who does the research and writing and raising of her subject.*

I won't realize it at the time, but these will be the burdens of everything I write: no time, no pay, and my motherhood—which gives me my material and insight—is working against me, professionally.

Barbara, whom I love, writes back: *Strong argument. Let me present it.*

But in the end, the managing editor decides the story will not be written by me. It will be written by a staff writer, by a guy.

———

The photographer arrives an hour early, so my hair, which I've recently cut short to my chin, is frizzy and half-damp, and I'm still wearing the old yellow sweater I'd thrown on after my shower. But Anna's beauty needs no preparation; she's wearing a green onesie and a navy-blue cable-knit headband. I play with her in the crunchy leaves in our sunny front yard. I place her on my chest and fly her above me in the air.

When the photographer is putting his things in the back of his car, he stops and says, "You know, my son has hearing loss, too."

"What?" I say, shocked.

"Yeah, they didn't catch it till he was in kindergarten."

"Did he have anything else going on?" I ask.

"He had some kidney issues," he says. And then: "He never had a diagnosis. He was only five pounds when he was born."

The journalist for *The Denver Post* comes the next day. His name is John, and he's incredibly attentive and kind. He also arrives unaware of how much I have to say. He sits wide-eyed in a chair, scribbling down notes, and asks me a few times to repeat myself. Lori, our ASL teacher, is there too, and we sit on the ground in front of the coffee table, signing with Anna who's now, at eighteen months, able to stand while holding on. I explain to John that Lori doesn't know the cause of her own deafness either, which was congenital but nongenetic—that it's statistically more likely to be CMV than anything else. After John is finished interviewing me, he leaves me to continue discussing things with a videographer named Lindsay, who is a mother of two girls the same ages as mine, and who will be accompanying me to an appointment I've made.

It's to see an MFM—a maternal-fetal medicine specialist—who will tell me just how active CMV still is in my body, in case I happen to become pregnant again.

The lobby at my MFM's office is decorated with minimalist sketches of women curved over their newborns, their bodies umbrella-like, natural shields. When I begin the paperwork for admission, I lean over and show Lindsay, who's filming, that there is, predictably, no mention on the intake packet for CMV. I will have to check "Other" and then explain our situation—though CMV is more common, of course, than every other risk I see there.

Before my exam, we sit with the MFM in a conference room to establish certain points for the film. The doctor listens intently without interrupting. She asks how Anna is doing, whether she has cochlear implants. When I'm finished talking, she tells me she's actually involved with a study on CMV—and for a second, I think I've misheard what she said.

She goes on, though, to explain the study's design. First, they've screened all the participating pregnant women for evidence of a recent CMV infection. Of the women who fit this profile, half will be randomly, unknowingly placed in a placebo group, and they will not receive any treatment. The other half will take an investigatory drug while pregnant called CytoGam, to see if it will help stop a mother's body from transmitting CMV infection to her fetus. (Eventually, the study will be canceled due to "futility"—the treatment doesn't seem to be working.)

The MFM is articulate, kind, and clearly knowledgeable about CMV. But there's something familiar, something nagging about this study's design. What about the women who had no evidence—either prior or current—of a CMV infection in their bodies at the beginning of the study?

These women are what's called seronegative—meaning they've never had any contact with CMV and therefore are at much higher risk of a primary infection, which again will reach the fetus about 35 percent of the time. Seronegative women would have been exited from the study, sent home to have a hopefully healthy pregnancy.

"I realize the seronegative women couldn't be involved in the study," I tell the MFM. "But before you turned them away, did you tell them how to avoid CMV for the rest of their pregnancies?"

"Actually," she says, thinking it over, "now that you mention it, no. No, I don't think we did."

7

In the mornings, before the girls are awake, I sit at my desk in the family room, which backs up to an L-shaped, built-in bookshelf. Behind me are mostly books by women, about women, and as time goes on, more and more of them are about pregnancy. Whether I'm at home or in a bookstore or at the library, I have a habit of searching the indexes of books like these for any mention of CMV, and I always feel a mixture of validation and deflation every time it doesn't appear.

CMV is not in *Mayo Clinic Guide to a Healthy Pregnancy*. It's not in Dr. Sears's *The Healthy Pregnancy Book*. It's not in *What to Expect When You're Expecting*. I'm hopeful that I'll find it in *Expecting Better*, Emily Oster's best seller whose subtitle reads, "Why the Conventional Pregnancy Wisdom Is Wrong—and What You *Really* Need to Know." Given Oster's detailed research as an economist and the book's 2014 publication date, I'm fairly certain I'll find CMV in the book. But I don't. The index jumps from "cord clamping" to "CVS."

Years later, when I email Emily Oster, who's a mother herself and a professor at Brown University, I ask her if she didn't know about CMV during the writing of *Expecting Better*. Was CMV left out of the book because she didn't know it existed? Or did she knowingly omit it because there wasn't enough data for her to mention the disease that outweighs all the others she covers? She writes back: "I had the experience of not having CMV mentioned until after publication. Even my medical editor on the book didn't raise it in editing. Which, in retrospect, I think is surprising."

This, of course, is much less surprising to me.

She does say she intends to include CMV in the next version of the book, but I think of the interim—of all the years people will read about the best practices of pregnancy and still not know about CMV.

Sitting at my desk, I can feel CMV's absence on my shelves. But I realize I also want to know if CMV is absent way before publication—in the classroom. Are therestudies quantifying how much (or how little) doctors are learning about CMV during medical school? I'm searching online for an answer when I find something else. It's a short video produced by Duke University, and in it, a professor named Kathleen Muldoon is speaking against a velvet blue backdrop.

"I am a medical educator, I am an anthropologist," she says, "and I am a CMV mommy now."

Kathleen has steady eyes and a bold haircut—shorter than her jaw, with textured dark brown bangs. She's easy to listen to, but intense. Kathleen explains that while teaching embryology for seven years, she never formally taught her medical students about congenital CMV. She had, of course, been familiar with TORCH screening (the test that Kate, the med student in Sitka, had referenced), so she knew CMV existed. But missing from Kathleen's lectures, which went into great detail about major disruptions to development, was the disease that outnumbered all the others—the disease with which her son would be born.

"It occurred to me as an anthropologist," Kathleen says in the video, "that our biases and the way we present information will actually form students' impressions of basic science, but also the clinical implications of basic science."

I've long understood, of course, that biases shape the decisions we make in the world. But until now I haven't considered that our biases about disease dictate, in many cases, whether a patient lives or dies, whether a disease is eliminated or continues to exist. I picture medical students' lecture halls around the country, how bereft they likely are of stories like Kathleen's, and how subconsciously biased and lacking their understanding of CMV might be.

I do find one study online, published in 2014, that assessed CMV knowledge in medical school students, and it concludes: "Significant knowledge gaps regarding transmission and treatment were observed in all medical school years."

It strikes me now that I've witnessed this lack of education myself. When Anna was born, my sister-in-law Taisa (pronounced Tye-EE-sah, she's Ukrainian) was a medical resident in family practice. Taisa had sat on my floor, lovingly holding Anna, while gently asking about her head size, her hearing tests, her weight. She didn't offer any suggestions, any mention of testing Anna for CMV, and then off to Alaska we went. But right after Anna's diagnosis, Taisa confessed to me on the phone: "I'm just kicking myself I didn't think of CMV. It crossed my mind. But I didn't know enough about it or think it was common enough for me to stop and think, *Maybe that's what Anna has.*"

Later Taisa will end up a physician at the hospital where Anna was born. And together we will address the diagnosis that is missing from every infant born still, small, or into silence in its halls.

———

When I email Kathleen, she tells me all the details, starting with her pregnancy: she had a toddler, her daughter Genevieve, when she became pregnant with her second child, Gideon. At the time, she was co-teaching alongside OBs and pediatricians at Dartmouth Hitchcock Hospital in New Hampshire and the risk of CMV never came up. When an ultrasound at twenty weeks showed that her baby had an echogenic bowel (a sign of CMV), her OB ordered a TORCH test, which did indicate Kathleen had long-term antibodies to CMV. Then Kathleen's doctor said she could order a more specific CMV antibody test, so she requested it and found out she had both long-term *and* short-term antibodies to CMV. But her doctor told her, incorrectly, that it would be impossible to pass the virus onto her child. And she believed him.

Later, on more frequent ultrasounds, the width of the baby's skull showed up small (another sign of CMV), but the doctor pointed at her husband, Seth, and said, "His head is kind of small, too."

When Gideon was born in 2013, he looked like any baby—a full head of dark hair, eyes alert, Apgar score good. But the OB who arrived to discharge Kathleen said, "Does he look a little jaundiced? Maybe we should put him under some lights." When they did, a mottled purple rash appeared out of nowhere. Then came the revelation that he had hepatosplenomegaly—a long medical term for enlarged liver and spleen. Kathleen calls this "the classic trio of CMV symptoms": jaundice, petechiae (rash), and hepatosplenomegaly. Gideon would end up severely disabled by congenital CMV: he has seventeen specialists and thirty-six diagnoses, which include cerebral palsy, epilepsy, hearing and vision loss, and developmental delays.

When I tell Kathleen I wish she lived closer because I'd love to meet her and Gideon—or really, any other child with CMV—she asks if I'm in the CMV Mommies Facebook group, and I about fall out of my chair.

———

I thought I'd searched for it. But maybe I'd typed *parents* or *mothers* instead of *mommies*. Entering the name correctly, I find it immediately. And once the admin grants me access, I'm obsessed.

Here are the people I knew existed but couldn't find. Here is CMV's wingspan, which is even wider than I'd conceived. Mothers arrive and speak from what seems like every socioeconomic bracket, race, and nation, posting comments from Poland, Mexico, and Ireland; Malta, South Korea, and England. Some are in Colorado Springs, Longmont, Denver, even Wheat Ridge! I'm moved by the compassion offered from opposite ends of the spectrum, from mothers who've lost their children to mothers who are currently appealing insurance decisions.

People here are honest, their faces and homes unmade. Medical equipment in the background hasn't been cleared for family photos; there's no romantically filtered sunset when someone posts a video of their child's difficult behavior or recurrent seizures. I see PT moves we aren't doing, a spandex swing I can buy for Zaley, ideas for the hell of putting Anna in the car or in any room lacking light. Most healing of all is that people have responses—a totally novel addition to my devastatingly answer-lacking CMV experience. *Does your child arch their back all the time?* I ask, and the comments all ping back within minutes: *Yes!* Or, *It's a vestibular thing.*

Some mothers don't know the basics of CMV and post questions like *How did I get CMV???* and *Talk to me abt Asymptomatic and Symptomatic!,* while other mothers summarize complex medical journals or rattle off virology facts like they have Ph.D.'s. The most vocal seem to be the mothers who ran in-home daycares or worked at group daycare centers while pregnant and never learned about CMV, even though having frequent contact with young children in these settings makes a woman five to twenty-five times more likely to contract CMV than women not in contact with young children. (Hospital workers, on the other hand, do not contract CMV as often because universal precautions against all bodily fluids are more standard in their field.)

A number of these mothers in the group have lost their children to congenital CMV and have been working to educate childcare providers by explaining simple tips: that after a diaper change, diaper wipes are not sufficient to remove CMV from the hands; nor is hand sanitizer as effective as washing your hands for fifteen seconds with soap and water. These parents are involved with legal change in many states because while OSHA (the Occupational Safety and Health Administration) characterizes CMV as a recognized hazard, there has never been any federally regulated policy to educate childcare workers about the risk of CMV.

The most responded-to conversation in the group, though, might be the one that's ignited when a *pregnant* woman is granted membership. They've either received results of short-term antibodies during pregnancy, or they've had an amniocentesis after twenty-one weeks—the only way to confirm the presence of CMV in their fetus. *My OB has suggested termination,* they ask, *but what do you suggest?*

I've watched as the vast majority of CMV moms in the group responded that their children with CMV have become the lights of their lives. No matter the responding mother's stance on abortion, no matter her financial situation, no matter the baby's prognosis, hundreds of CMV moms have replied with photos of their children— ones who are in wheelchairs with cerebral palsy, ones who have cochlear implants and autism, and a striking number of children who weren't affected at all by CMV who are hiking and swimming and zooming past the camera on scooters, despite testing positive for CMV in utero and their doctors' dire predictions that they'd be a "vegetable for the rest of their lives."

It seems to me that these exchanges are more about a woman's capacity to handle unexpected challenges than about the value of any child's life. And most of the mothers in the group are clear: this won't be easy, but yes you can handle it. One of my favorite lines from a CMV mom whose daughter has brain damage and hearing loss is: "Would never ever replace her for a baby with no issue never." One mother writes: "It is a lot of work having a medically complex child, and I wish I could have a conversation with him, but he is so worth it." She also cautions the pregnant mothers in the audience: "Know that doctors often don't see the joys of complex children, just the medical burden."

Of course, posting pictures of smiling disabled children and attesting to their joy has the potential to simplify the very complex issue of paying for their care, and there is far too little therapeutic and monetary support, in most states, for families and caretakers of disabled children—a point many mothers make in the group. But the lack of available funding for those with disabilities is implicated in a vicious cultural cycle that denies their value to society: until we say that these kids are worth having, there will be far fewer of them and therefore less support for them and their parents.

———

Reading these exchanges sends me, as always, to the medical journals to see whether having the CMV discussion with pregnant women might increase the number of abortions women have—often due to uninformed fear or misunderstanding. I find one study, conducted in Italy in 2007, in which a team including Dr. Tiziana Lazzarotto set out to measure the opposite: might terminations decrease if women are more expertly counseled about CMV?

In the study, all the women had evidence of short-term antibodies during pregnancy and were then divided into two groups: group 1 consisted of women whose antibody tests indicated they had a primary infection, putting them at the highest risk of transmitting CMV to the fetus. Group 2, on the other hand, consisted of women who had evidence of long-term antibodies, too, and thus were probably experiencing a nonprimary infection and were very unlikely to transmit CMV to their fetuses.

In Lazzarotto's study, most of the women had already been

advised by their own referring doctors to seek termination, no matter
if they had a primary or a nonprimary infection. The study assumed
that women with any evidence of a recent CMV infection would
opt to terminate about 12 percent of the time—that is, if they didn't
understand the specifics of CMV.

But unlike in the real world, in the Italian study, all the participants were provided with thorough explanations of congenital CMV.
The women with suspected primary infections were counseled about
fetal risks, the advisability of ultrasound monitoring (since a large
number of these babies will end up having no abnormalities), and
the possibility of diagnosing fetal infection with certainty later, by
amniocentesis.

In the nonprimary group, the women were assured that there
was a low risk of fetal damage and that ultrasound monitoring alone
would suffice as an alternative to the more invasive testing of an
amniocentesis.

In the end, fifty-three of the women, or 11.9 percent, in the primary infection group ended up terminating (thus, the authors' ret-
roactive assumption about how many women, in general, would
likely abort in the absence of counseling). But only five women, or
0.4 percent, ended up terminating in the nonprimary infection group.
Lazzarroto's results, which were published in the *American Journal of
Obstetrics and Gynecology*, were shocking: when women were counseled by an expert physician about CMV and thoroughly understood
their risk, abortions were reduced by 73 percent.

———

When I turn away from my research, I am desperate again for pictures of babies. Looking at them in the CMV Mommies group, I
realize I've done a 180-degree turn from when I first scrolled through
the National CMV Foundation's stories; now I want to see all the
babies with CMV, and I'm here without fear.

I swear I love these children the first time I see them. Whether
they're visibly afflicted or without outward sign, I love them because
I love Anna, because the presence of CMV in their bodies makes me
want to fight for them. Because they are—or they were, at least for
a time—a living, contributing force in this world.

I'm relieved when I read another mom, Kimberly's, similar sentiment:

> *Can I say something slightly creepy? I love your kids. I mean, I love them to the point that I cry when you post that they're hurt or sick. I laugh and feel joy when you have good news. I feel like I've somehow got hundreds of babies all over the world who have mamas and daddies, but are still mine.*

Another day, a mom named Andrea posts a picture of her son who's two, has cerebral palsy, and wears cochlear implants: *Axel just said the "Buh" sound for the first time ever!!!!! AHHHH!!! I am in total shock!*

I don't believe I've ever seen a mother this excited about the sound of the letter *B*—or any of her child's milestones, really.

Maybe it's for the better that these moms and their babies are protected from me by distance and difficult car rides. By the third photo that another CMV child's parents have posted, I feel I know them, I wish we lived closer, I want to have everyone over.

———

And then a CMV mother does just that: she asks if the girls and I want to come to her house for coffee. She has two boys who are roughly the same age as my girls. Her name is Erin; she's a lawyer, and so is her husband. She read some of my writing online, on my blog. Hearing from Erin makes me realize it was myself I was rescuing just as much as any other CMV mom who might feel alone. I wrote that blog because I wanted to be found.

When the girls and I arrive at their house, Erin is standing in the doorway with her older son, Michael, who is Zaley's age. Erin has blond hair, is wearing exercise clothes, and is remarkably thin. I wonder if stress does the same thing to her body as it does to mine—takes part of me away. When she shakes my hand, she's stronger than I expected. Her smile is genuine, her teeth a bright white.

Erin steps aside to let us in, and her house is large and clean. There's hand sanitizer in two places, in sight. I know she's acutely aware of viruses now, like me. I also see a little baby sitting inside a laundry basket padded with clothes—a common trick moms use for low-toned kids. This is Matthew, her child with CMV.

I've actually seen Matthew before. When his hearing aids were activated, Ashton Kutcher—a disability advocate—shared the video on Facebook, and it went viral. I'm not surprised it got so many views; Matthew has giant blue eyes and peach-fuzz blond hair, and in the video, his eyes nearly pop out of their sockets, he's so excited about sound. He's over one year old now. He can't yet crawl.

But when Erin takes him out, the way he moves is incredibly cute. He's like a little Roomba—those cordless vacuums that scoot around the house, spinning and finding corners before they turn around and find another place to go. She barely has to keep an eye on him while the older kids demand snacks and things to do. He just scoots and rolls, under tables, through the dining room, past us into the kitchen. He isn't on his hands or knees yet, but he travels far, and he does it soundlessly, happily.

We stand at the counter and talk. We sit on the couch and cry. Before I leave, Erin says she and Jeff are going to meet with a senator about enacting a CMV bill in Colorado, and do I want to come with them? Of course, I cry again.

If Sitka—and life itself—have affirmed any cliché, it's that when it rains, it pours. And so on the same day that I get an email from my MFM stating that my CMV titres indicate it's safe to try for another baby (which tends to be about a year after you've had a child with congenital CMV), I also get an email from *The New York Times* "Well" editor. She wants to publish my short essay on CMV.

With Anna in my arms, I rush into Luke's office. When I tell him about the publication, he stands up to hug and congratulate me. And because he's so proud of me, I figure I have an opening. With his ear against mine, I say: "Want to have another baby?"

PART V

CARETAKING

"Sorrow is assuaged by bodily remedies."

SAINT THOMAS AQUINAS

I

———

When raisins taste like Band-Aids and coffee loses its allure, I know.

"I'm sure I'm pregnant," I say to Luke, who's pouring his own coffee at the kitchen counter.

"Did you take a test?" he asks, sliding the carafe back into the machine.

"It was negative. But I'm sure." I always know before the pink cross shows up on the stick.

He sets down his coffee cup and holds up both hands. He's counting on his fingers, counting down the months.

"So late October . . . early November?" he says with hope.

"It'll be close, but yes."

I know he's counting past fishing season to first rifle season in mid-October, when he'll be hunting with all his brothers and his dad.

Hunting and fishing, of course, aren't more important to Luke than me or our kids. In fact, Luke always says he'd be fine if he never shot an elk again. And he means it: he hunts more to be with other people in the wilderness than to harvest anything from it. And now that we have kids to go with him, he wants to preserve the legacy of the wild for them—to give them a story that starts with knowledge, necessitates patience, and involves paying close attention in the silence. In this, we are not so different.

This time, this pregnancy, the timing feels right, like I might even deliver with Luke in the room. I'm tingling and excited and optimistic. I also know we only have about a week before morning sickness turns me into my alter ego.

"Let's get away," I tell him.

So Luke calls his parents, and they agree to take the girls for a few days while we stay at their place in the mountains.

———

The cabin is only an hour's drive from our house. It has vaulted ceilings with beams salvaged from a homestead in Montana and a big stone hearth, where Luke makes a roaring fire and feeds it till we go to bed. We wake late, eat egg sandwiches, read books on the floor in front of the flames. We talk about the kids and how glorious life must have been before we had them, even though we know it was just as full of desire and malaise. In the afternoons, we fly fish in the Blue River as carpets of snow cushion the wintry valley. Afterward I swim laps at the Silverthorne Rec Center, and Luke sits in the hot tub, waving at me like a lazy pink crab between sets.

The mountains make me more contemplative, and so does the pool. While I go back and forth, I think about the flip-turn CMV put into my life. I think about how I intend to take better care of my body this time, knowing that there's also no such thing as a zero-risk pregnancy—that life, disability, the unexpected, whatever you want to call it, finds a way.

But once we're home and the nausea arrives, I have unrealistic expectations of all my family members. I snap at the kids when they drop drinks by accident. I yell at Luke when he fails to tell me he needs to leave for church an hour earlier than usual to help set up the baptismal font for someone else's baby. I resent that his generosity means I'm silently bearing the heavier load. I know humility means swallowing this kind of tit for tat, but humility is a bar set too high for me right now.

I cycle between my MFM and the optimistic OBs at the same practice where I was seen for my pregnancy with Anna—the only clinic anywhere near our house that will take my insurance, even though it doesn't seem fair that this place, where I have such a history, is my only reasonable option. During my first ultrasound, I cringe when the OB says, "Everything looks great"—the same thing the providers always said about Anna in utero, till the very end. I realize that I'm almost hoping for something irregular—to have the sighting, the closure, the naming that, with Anna, I never had. Instead, it's all good: the rounded tip of the nose, the thumb aiming for the mouth, the hardworking chambers of the heart.

At one of my early appointments, I see the OB I'd spoken to over the phone when I was in Sitka—the one who'd said women don't want to worry about one more thing. I ask him if he's placed any CMV brochures around the office, since I'd told him they were available for free on the National CMV website. He says no, but if I fax one over, he'll have a look. I wonder who in the world still owns a fax.

"By the way," he says, "it's impossible for you to have another baby with CMV."

This is neither correct nor answers any question I asked.

I've already talked to Dr. Suresh Boppana again, who has studied CMV in women all over the world, and he told me that it's not actually impossible. But yes, my chances of having a second baby with CMV are very very low, around 0.001 percent. While most cases of congenital CMV around the world are due to nonprimary infections (from encountering a new strain of CMV or CMV reactivating in a woman's system), a CMV mother having another child with congenital CMV would be kind of like getting struck by lightning twice.

"The good news," Dr. Boppana told me, "is that if you've already had a baby with congenital CMV, you're much more protected than any other woman who's pregnant or trying to conceive."

But I feel more vulnerable than ever. Not because of CMV but because I believe a typical pregnancy might be hiding something else that's understudied, undisclosed. When I get the flu, I lie on our pink couch, where I'd been sick with Anna developing inside me, and I Google dangerous infections that can transmit during the first trimester of pregnancy. When I don't see CMV, the searing hot-cold of my rage reignites.

At every appointment, I'm disappointed that even after I tell my doctors I'm writing a book, they don't want to hear the story. No one ever asks me how I'm feeling to be pregnant again, what it felt like, what happened before.

Not sure where to put my knowledge, I start leaving CMV flyers at OB offices, silently, around town.

The months pass in a dizzying mixture of misery and delight. One night Zaley is singing to my belly in the bathtub and asks me if the baby can hear her. I tell her the truth no one ever says: some babies can and some babies can't. I'm so nauseous I want to be in a coma for the next two months, and yet my children are more interesting than ever. Anna thinks she has a baby in her tummy, too, and she puffs out her stomach, slaps it with both palms, and says, "See? Baby?"

Our OT, Leslie, comes over and shows me how to put Anna's walking braces comfortably on her feet. The braces are thick pieces of plastic that fit her arches perfectly because they're shaped from molds we had made in Alaska. They're a girly camouflage print, all gradations of pink. Her socks go on first, then the braces, which Velcro over the bridge of each foot. They need to be tight. They encase her feet, her ankles, and her lower calves before she puts on her shoes (none of which fit over the braces, so my friend Mia brings over a pair of her girls' Pumas, two sizes too big, and they work).

When Anna is nineteen months old, she starts taking one step at a time. I wipe the tears from my eyes every time this happens the first few days. Then one night, completely unannounced, just before she turns two, Anna stands up in her braces and sprints, bowlegged, all the way to Luke, who is sitting across the room. Zaley is standing next to me when it happens, and she starts screaming and jumping with glee.

"Where did that COME from?" she shrieks.

It's like Anna has been saving up this triumphant reveal—one more piece of her lifelong secret.

I never post Anna's steps to the CMV Mommies group online, because I've been on the other side of this kind of pride. Over the summer Mia and her husband had bought the house across the street from ours in Colorado, and one day when Anna was not yet crawling, Mia texted me a video of her daughter, Anna's exact age, *running* around our yard. She meant nothing by it—just total excitement to be neighbors—but I told Mia: it hurt.

Now I have a child who's running, and other people don't, even if the way Anna's body moves is due to no fault or effort of our own. Our ability to exchange media today can draw stark contrasts visible only to the more sensitive of the two sides. It's like when parents of typical kids post dramatic black and white pictures on social media of their child in an ER for a reason they purposely don't disclose (and later, in the comments, reveal it to be a minor sprain of the wrist). When I see, on the same day, a post from a CMV parent about their child being airlifted for seizures that won't stop, I recognize that some people genuinely need support and others simply want attention. There is a difference.

For Lent this year, I decide I'll delete the Facebook app on my phone for a while, see how silence feels instead.

For us, Lent is intense. Every Friday night for six weeks leading up to Easter, we have a lengthy service that lasts way past the kids' bedtimes. It is dark, candlelit, and full of a long silence, during which we lie facedown on the floor. Most years during Lent, I can feel the dimness of the season upon my heart. But that doesn't mean I dislike it. Lent is when I'm most intentional about my choices, when I try to get up before the kids, to be still for ten minutes, to think about the better way I haven't been.

For forty days, we also fast from meat (unless I'm pregnant or nursing, so I almost always have a dispensation) and whatever other habits we choose to forgo. Unlike what I'd always assumed as a child when we proudly told our classmates what we were giving up for Lent, I've learned that fasting was never intended to be a practice of outward piety. Fasting from physical things is actually a training tool for the harder things we can't fully teach ourselves: abstaining from things like anxiety, irritability, and fury (an abstinence I could currently use).

In the Eastern Catholic and Orthodox churches, Lent starts with my favorite service of the year: it's on Sunday evening, as the light is falling, and it's called Vespers of Forgiveness. It's brief and quiet but profoundly moving. The entire community lines up in one long line. Then the first person in the line—typically the priest—stands in front of the first community member and says, "Forgive me," then that person's name. Then that person says, "Forgive me, Father," in response. Then both people prostrate to each other, which means they kneel down in front of each other, placing their foreheads on the ground in a gesture of sorrow and penance. The priest asks forgiveness of every person in the church as they are asking it of him. And as he's going along, the second person is following him, asking forgiveness of every person and receiving it, and then the third person follows, and the fourth, and so on, until by the end of the service, the line has reversed itself and everyone now stands in forgiveness of one another.

I'm always amazed by how personal this practice feels. When you meet the eyes of each person, you think of all the ways you may have hurt them, all the ways they may have hurt you. When you say *forgive me,* it carries a culpability and a desperation. What moves me most deeply is when I think of what I'm asking of my children. *Forgive me, Zaley, for expecting too much of you. Forgive me, Anna, for not fully protecting you.*

As one of my friends says of anyone experiencing Vespers of Forgiveness for the first time, "You come back, or you think, *I never want to be that close or accountable again.*"

After thirty prostrations and a heavier uterus than usual, my thighs and knees quake. I feel a rawness of spirit I can't quite explain.

"Forgive me, Luke," I say to my husband.

"Forgive me, Megan," he says to me.

"Forgive me, Zaley," I say to my daughter.

"Forgive me, Mom," she says back.

And then Anna stands in front of me, wordless, then bows her tiny little body to the floor.

2

The next vespers service we have is in Alaska. I'm twenty-four weeks pregnant, we've just landed, and I'd rather stay home, to be honest— order Kenny's Wok, watch a movie, put the kids to bed early. But Luke is the only tenor in town, and because he's been away from us for the last six weeks, he really wants us to come.

Going to church for me is like exercising; I'm never thrilled at the idea, but I always leave a little stronger than when I went in. There's also a sense of excitement tonight: there's a new priest behind the Byzantine iconostasis—an image-clad wall that blocks the altar from view. We know the new priest is Native Alaskan, that he and his family just moved to Sitka from a tiny village out beyond the Aleutian chain. We've also heard he has a lot of kids, and I'm eager for someone else's kids to be louder than ours in church.

Luke is warming up with the choir to the right of the altar, and the girls and I are in the back on an aged, upholstered pew. When the door opens from the street, I can hear the rain showering over the old wooden buildings downtown, feel the cold damp air rushing in through the door. When I turn around to see who has entered, I know it must be the priest's wife because I've never seen her before.

Her face is heart-shaped, and she has tight, youthful skin. She looks both approachable and slightly intimidating. Her black eyes have a readiness, some unblinking expectancy. She's wearing a heads-carf, a long skirt, and tennis shoes. Behind her, I count the children approaching the nave: one, two, three, four, five. Then their young-est child, their sixth, who looks like he's about three, comes running down the maroon carpet into the center of the church before stop-ping, hockey style, with a huge, mostly toothless grin on his face.

And in a town in Alaska that has never contained any deaf children besides our own, I see this child has two flashing green lights on his head. I sign as discreetly as I can to Luke, across the church, *See him? See that boy's ears??*

Father and Michelle's youngest son, Theophan—which means "God appearing"—has cochlear implants.

———

Theophan does not have CMV. At his family's home, over a dinner I can't stomach of seal oil, walrus, and transparent herring eggs suspended in water and clinging to a branch—which Zaley consumes by the handful, with zeal—we learn that Theophan contracted meningitis when he was four months old, which caused profound deafness in both of his ears. Theophan doesn't speak at all; he uses sign.

When I stand up to get a glass of water in the long ranch home provided to the Andrews family by the Orthodox church, Theophan follows me into the kitchen. He's a little bit upset. He's waving and stomping at me to get me to understand. *Shoes!* He signs, vigorously. *You have shoes on! Shoes go over there!*

I sign *I'm sorry*, and he leads me by the hand to the mud room, where thirty-some pairs of shoes are arranged in neat, double-decker lines. I'm totally impressed by Theophan's logic and emphasis. And I should have known: wearing shoes beyond the entryway is an Alaskan sin.

There's a noticeable quiet in the Andrews' home, even though they have more kids than most of our friends. The children, for the most part, do their own thing. They eat at the table, but they leave it when they're finished—unlike at our house, where we're constantly negotiating the next bite, the ability to be excused. A few of their older kids are on their phones or watching a movie in the family room. No one rushes to the help a younger child who's whining or bickering. Michelle and Father seem utterly relaxed, almost oblivious to the fact that there are now eight kids walking around with red popsicles on their carpet.

The Andrews are Yup'ik, a Native tribe of Alaskans, whose name comes from the word *yuk* meaning "person" plus *pik* which means "real." They are *real people*. Later my friend Peter will explain that there's no small talk among the Yup'ik—this would be fake. They don't say anything that doesn't need to be said. They find the filling of silence useless and exhausting. I, on the other hand, am asking question after question about Theophan, which Michelle answers happily but with as few words as she needs.

When they do communicate, Father and Michelle use a mixture of sign language and English and Yup'ik, a guttural language with a lot of fricatives—clicking noises most white people can't make with the underused muscles in their throat. (Father and Luke are already making a game of saying as many Yup'ik phrases as they can with fricatives that sound like they have the F-word in them.) In the hours we're at their house—and later, over the course of many years—I find a peace in their peace, in the lack of obligation to speak.

It's not like we sit in silence, either; we discuss all sorts of things— how they're going to build a *maqivik* (a dry steam house) in their yard, how much moose an uncle in the village is sending next month, how much mayonnaise Father likes on his rice. Their daughter who's Zaley's age has a deadpan look like her mom. Zaley takes to her immediately, tempered by her confidence and calm. There are rarely arguments between the kids. And I never once hear Michelle raise her voice.

I assume, in the moment, that this is because we are guests. But later I'll find out that Yup'ik mothers never, ever yell at their kids; scolding children is viewed as deeply immature by their culture, a sign that an adult can't control themselves. Silence is the opposite.

———

After dinner, Michelle and I sit on a white couch chatting and watching the kids. On the wall above us are clothing items of each of her children's that she's pinned to the wall—"It cuts down on noise," she explains—and I ask her if it's been hard for her to figure out all of Theophan's needs in a town like Sitka. She looks at me kind of like she doesn't know what I'm asking, having come from a village of three hundred, then she says, "Oh, sometimes," as though she's not been tasked with anything out of the ordinary. She does explain her frustrations with the school system, says she's working with the Anchorage School for the Deaf to provide a deaf educator for him in town. But then she says, with the sharpness returning to her eyes that I saw in church: "It's an honor to be his parents."

Besides not yelling, Michelle seldom tells her children not to do what they're doing. Especially Theophan, who can be loud and frantic—and has no awareness of personal space—which I find totally endearing. (At one point, he clambers into my lap and turns my head with both hands toward him to make sure I'm paying attention to his signs.) Two of their boys are in middle school, and one of them is aggravating the other one endlessly, ripping his feet out from under him and ruffling his hair. Michelle simply gives them a look, and the boys push each other outside. There are no apologies for their behavior, no mention of behaviors at all.

The journalist Michaeleen Doucleff writes about another arctic Indigenous tribe, the Inuit, who approach parenting similarly. These parents believe, as Doucleff puts it, that "there's no race to acquire emotional maturity." What a perfect skill set, I realize, for raising a child with disabilities.

And what a humane, self-caring approach to the act of parenting, too. Father and Michelle's quiet way doesn't impart patience to me, exactly—that will always be hard for me, a lifetime's worth of work. But it gives me *permission* to step back and let things be a mess, to excuse myself from the goal-oriented, achievement-clawing "mommy wars" that have so defined my experience of motherhood.

———

It may be that Father and Michelle have a more mature understanding of parenting than I do, having learned to be parents from their parents and their parents before them who never left the village—a subarctic stretch, as flat as a stamp, in the pictures they show us, proud of home. There are ATVs and fish-drying racks and weathered canoes hauled up on a desolate beach. There is no entitlement here.

In the village, they tell me, they ran a crisis pregnancy center. I wonder, of course, if they've heard of congenital CMV, especially since, like Black children, Native American children with CMV have double the mortality rate of white children born with the disease. When I tell them about CMV, they are silent, nodding, taking it in.

"I can't believe we didn't know," Michelle says. Then they are silent again.

Later, when I tell Luke I envy this family's ability to keep calm, he explains to me that a central tenet of Orthodox prayer is working toward a profound inner silence—or *hesychia*—as a way of curing the soul of all kinds of noise, from anxiety to insecurity to mental and even physical illness. *Hesychia* brings a person closer to the essence of God—an essence that, according to Orthodoxy, can never fully be known—and *hesychia* is reached through a stillness of spirit and an abandonment of sensory things, even *the senses.*

Which is maybe why later, when I ask Father if they'd like to send Theophan with us to Colorado, just temporarily, to meet some other deaf children at RMDS, to see our audiologist and our AVT, Father says no—they would suffer too greatly without him. Theophan is one of their greatest gifts.

The rest of the summer races. It rains less than usual. We go out less than usual, too, because my pelvis feels like it might break in half. But two things happen that change my life.

The first is when Luke walks in one day after fishing for halibut, offshore, and says:

"You won't believe this. This guy Örn"—pronounced *Ern*—"was on my boat today. He fished with me twelve years ago. Great guy, Icelandic, crazy smart. Today he told me he works for a startup company in Massachusetts that works on vaccines."

"What's it called?" I ask.

"His company's called Moderna, Inc.," Luke says.

"Never heard of it," I say back. (The pandemic is still years away.)

"Me either. But get this: when I told Örn our daughter was born with a congenital disease called CMV, he stopped reeling, looked at me, and said: 'I'm the head of formulations for Moderna's CMV vaccine.'"

"Do you have his phone number?" I ask Luke, jittery.

"Yeah," Luke says. "I told him you'd be calling."

---

236 | Megan Nix

The next evening I'm parked outside the smoothie shop with a notebook in my hand when I dial the Massachusetts phone number to reach Örn.

He answers right away. "I'm on a long drive!" he says, in an accent that's energetic and charming. "Which is good, because we have a lot to talk about!"

For the next hour, he tries to explain in laymen's terms the way an mRNA vaccine works. "Basically, the technology tells your body, *Here's this Trojan horse of a virus*, so that next time, when your body meets that disease in the real world, it thinks, *You're not that big of a deal; I don't need to launch a huge response because I've already battled you before.*"

I scribble down phrases and descriptions as quickly as I can on the notebook balanced between the steering wheel and my chest. (The smoothie shop's blenders are too loud, the library's too quiet, and the kids at home are too loud, as well.) Örn tells me that when he joined Moderna in 2013, the company was really focused on rare disease treatments rather than vaccines. But in 2016, they started working on a CMV vaccine for women of childbearing age that would end up being successful at producing an antibody response in the body that neutralizes the virus and prevents infection. (Of course, this fully synthetic mRNA platform is the same technology that the company will later replicate to prevent severe COVID-19.) The CMV vaccine will also end up further ahead than any of the other projects at Moderna prior to the pandemic, even though it will never receive any government funding. The project is investor-funded only, led by a conviction that CMV is a disease that disables children, significantly contributes to stillbirth and infant mortality, and shouldn't exist.

Örn mentions that years ago, it was Moderna's CEO, Stéphane Bancel, who suggested the company should address CMV because he knew the silent toll it was taking on women's pregnancies and he had two daughters who'd probably want to have kids. Later Stéphane will tell me this is true—and he was also compelled by the fact that for the last twenty years, all the big pharmaceutical companies had tried to make CMV vaccines and failed. "We thought mRNA science should be able to deal with the complexity of the virus. So we thought we had a responsibility to give it our best shot." This is one of the only times I've ever heard a public figure call CMV their "responsibility."

Örn is fully aware that the American public knows barely anything about CMV, which includes people who work with him. So after our call, he connects me with Moderna's public relations team to help educate their staff about congenital CMV.

When I pull up the Zoom meeting on my computer, three biotech geniuses in Boston are staring at me from the screen. "Tell us your story," one of them says. I can barely speak.

———

The other thing that happens takes place in a matter of seconds. I'm at the library for a few hours while a babysitter is watching the kids, and I'm walking toward the glass-walled conference room I've been reserving to write, when my friend Hannah exits that room through its transparent door.

Hannah is a filmmaker who knows how the creative world works—how it breaks your heart, takes over your mind, makes you feel like an imposter, makes you who you are. When I tell her that I'm working, very slowly, on a book about Anna and CMV, she says I should send my work to a literary agent, to someone in New York. I tell her I have so much to do—plus, I've done that before.

"Send it out," Hannah says, resolute. "Send it to the best agent you can find. The worst they can say is no."

"But it's not done," I tell her. "It's not even close."

"That's okay," she says. "Maybe they'll like what you've done so far. And maybe they'll pay you to write the rest."

Hannah is talking about an *advance*: the magic thing every writer wants to receive. An advance is when a publishing house takes a risk on you—paying you, up front, your share of whatever they think you'll make back. They are paying you to write.

I stop myself from even thinking about compensation for my time. And when Hannah leaves, I'm so hopped up on the idea of querying an agent, I can't sit down and write, either. So I walk across the street, around the Orthodox church in the center of downtown, and into my favorite store in Sitka: Old Harbor Books. They always have the local writers' books on a table in front of the door. To the right is the little nook for children, to the left is the new books section.

I walk left. I pick up a new book by a famous writer I love. I look at her acknowledgments, at the agent she has thanked.

I know this agent is far too powerful to represent someone like me. But Hannah's encouragement echoes through my head. At home, at night, I begin working in earnest on the opening chapters of my book.

3

Back in Colorado, we smoke our summer-caught salmon for Anna's therapists, drag the bassinet up from the basement, and buy butt cream and diapers for the new baby. Then it's my due date. That Sunday, because Father Chrysostom is out of town, we decide we'll go to a Roman Catholic church called St. Bernadette's, where we've never been as a family before, but where I have happy memories as a child.

My dad played the organ at St. Bernadette's thirty years ago, and on sleepy Saturday afternoons when my brothers went to their soccer games with my mom, I used to ride with him to church and listen while he played the pipe organ below the stained-glass windows of the saints. Now St. Bernadette's is only a few miles from our house. Luke's brother Brant and his wife, Annie, live even closer to St. Bernadette's, and they're going to meet us with their two little kids for mass.

We pile frantically out of our cars in the parking lot—a common scene among Luke's side of the family: late for church, with lots of blond kids, whose dads all look like clones. In between our cars, Annie places a hand on the shelf of my stomach and asks how I'm doing. That's when I have my first big contraction. I bend over at the hips and inhale.

"Are you in *labor?*" she asks, her hands gripping my shoulders, her eyes on the verge of laughter.

"Maybe," I tell her, knowing I am. "Let's go inside."

The church is divided into a front section of pews, an open space, then a back section of pews. We sit in the first row of the back section, so the whole front half of the congregation is in view. And immediately I get chills: the front half of the church is Deaf. I know because they're all signing that Sunday's psalm with their hands.

It turns out, St. Bernadette's is the largest Catholic church west of the Mississippi that enables the full participation of the Deaf community, with a priest who's fluent in ASL and says the entire mass in SimCom on Sundays.

When we reach the Alleluia, everyone in front of me raises their fist in the handshape for the letter *A,* which they wave around to the rhythm of the hymn. My eyes well up with tears. Annie looks at me and promptly looks away so she doesn't cry, too. I put my tongue to the roof of my mouth, point out the Deaf people to Anna, make her hand into the shape of an *A.* When Zaley isn't whispering to her cousin Clara, I see she's trying to sing and sign along.

At the end of mass, the girls want to have doughnuts, but I tell Annie we'd better go.

"Call us as soon as you head to the hospital!" she says, in that thrilled way other people are for a woman about to give birth—way more excited, way less terrified than the mother herself.

———

At midnight, I shake Luke awake and tell him we need to go *now.* Mia's husband, Jeremy, walks across the street to stay with the sleeping girls till my parents can make it to our house.

At the hospital, I earn myself a room. Even though this is a different baby, the pain is exactly the same: I always have back labor, and it feels like a flaming chainsaw is grinding through my hips from behind. I make a quick decision and say to the nurse, "Find the doctor with the needle, immediately."

The anesthesiologist is my hero. When he inserts the needle through a taped-up square on my spine, it feels like a fly landing on my back compared to the pain of contracting. A few minutes later I can breathe—I can even speak. Luke pours himself a cup of coffee, and then, true to form, falls asleep. The nurse says I should nap, too, and places a peanut-shaped ball between my legs to help the baby descend. I should call for her when I feel "uncomfortable."

I doze for an hour, then the discomfort is there, like a heaviness that must be released. I call for the nurse. She comes in with the midwife, who checks me and says it's time to push. I push. I push some more. I tell Luke that I really want to keep pushing. Luke—who hates labor and loves babies—says, "Okay, I know you can do it. But I'll just stay right up here, near your head."

I end up pushing for three hours.

The nurse suggests we summon the on-call OB.

When he strides in, he looks at me and stops in the middle of the room.

"Oh!" he says. "Hello!" He's the doctor who doesn't want to worry women, who told me it's impossible to have another baby with CMV.

I can tell he remembers me. I can tell he wants to deliver this baby without rolling me down to the bad place with knives.

Vespers of Forgiveness flashes in my mind, both of us in this vulnerable position, me thinking, *Forgive me for resenting you,* and maybe, just maybe, he's thinking something like *Forgive me for underestimating you.*

"Usually in this case, we'd be heading to the OR," he says. "But before we do that, I want to try one more thing. Are you okay with me trying a vacuum?"

I nod, in favor of anything to prevent surgery. So the midwife readies the tool—which I'd pictured as a high-power, sucker-outer like a vacuum at a car wash, but it's basically a small white funnel. He presses it against the baby's head, and immediately I feel the bulb inside me give. The doctor does, too. He turns to my midwife and says the most wonderful words: "Get dressed for delivery."

When I push the baby out of me, I first see the wondrous engineering of the blue and white cord. Then the same dark hair as Anna's. Then a face as wide as Zaley's. And then I hear it—the sound I've been imagining, the sound that either shocks you out of your prior existence or shocks you with its absence: the baby is screaming. The baby is big. The baby looks healthy. Luke squeezes my hand and says, "She's a girl."

The nurse cleans her, wraps her, brings her back. I tuck my new daughter inside my stretchy nightgown and feel her heat, her steady breath. She rests so motionlessly, I keep craning my neck to see if she's alive.

"Should we name her Naomi?" I ask Luke, after the woman who

called the *hesed* forth from Ruth. He says yes.

When I put my mouth to her ear and say her name, her head twitches on my chest, and I think instantly of Anna: how she was born silent and into silence; how she was fighting something as soon as she left me.

Luke knows what I'm thinking. He says, "She hears you, Meg. She's a beauty, isn't she?"

It's November 7. It's our anniversary.

The next day I know there's something I need to do. I ask the pediatrician on rotation from Children's Hospital to test Naomi for CMV.

She refuses.

Anna is in the room, sitting on the cushioned bench under the window. You can see the green lights of her cochlear implants reflecting off the glass, the pink plastic of her foot braces underneath her adaptive Nike FlyEase shoes that zip open from the back.

I point to Anna. "My daughter there, she has congenital CMV. I want to know."

"Give me five minutes," the pediatrician says, then leaves the room. When she comes back, she says: "I checked with my attending. Honestly, we both agree—it's just so rare, we don't see any reason to test."

It's in this moment, sitting in the hospital room with my child who has CMV and my infant who is unethically refused the option of being tested for the same *contagious* disease, that I feel a hot white rage, a rock solid conviction that something big and concrete has to change.

A few days later, at the pediatrician's office, I ask a nurse if they'll test Naomi for CMV. "Of course we will," she says. "Why wouldn't we?" She tapes the potty purse to Naomi, but I wait and wait, and she will not pee. When the nurse comes to check on us, she says Naomi can just wear the bag home, and I can bring it back.

A much faster, more convenient test is actually available, where a nurse or doctor can simply swab the inside of a newborn's cheek for

CMV, as long as they haven't just nursed. (CMV can be present in breastmilk, and you don't want the saliva swab contaminated by the mother's own fluids and yield a false positive, while the baby itself is uninfected. And despite the possibility of CMV being present in a mother's milk, it is always recommended for her to breastfeed, unless the baby was born under three pounds or before thirty weeks.) The newborn's saliva specimen is then expedited to a national reference laboratory in Utah called ARUP, where a laboratory assay—or test—is performed to detect CMV in a baby's DNA.

Two days after I bring the potty purse back to the pediatrician, the test results come back, and even though I knew what they'd be, I still feel a deep shiver of relief: Naomi is negative for congenital CMV.

———

There's a boy in Zaley's class named Leo whose mother is a labor and delivery nurse at Lutheran. Lauren is her name. At preschool drop-off, Lauren is always carrying her daughter Penelope, who's the same age as Anna—and, she looks like she's the same size as Anna. One day Lauren tells me Penelope was also born five pounds, full term. She has some challenges with eating, some motor delays. She, too, was born at Lutheran. And she was never tested for congenital CMV.

When I ask Lauren if she'll check and see how Lutheran usually processes tests for CMV, she says she will.

A few days later, Lauren texts me: *You're going to be mad. I don't think the lab at Lutheran has ever received a test for congenital CMV.*

———

Ever since Anna was diagnosed, I've been hesitant to involve my sister-in-law Taisa in my fight against CMV. It seemed, in the beginning, that it was my journey alone, and that to implicate a new doctor, at her first hospital of employment, in a controversial topic, could compromise her reputation—even her career.

But between Anna's birth and Naomi's, Taisa's mom underwent a kidney transplant for a rare genetic condition. While recovering from her transplant surgery, Taisa's mom almost died from a dangerous latent virus that likely reactivated while she was severely immunosuppressed. That virus was CMV.

CMV's medical dismissal had been important to Taisa before her mother was compromised by it. But now it seems even more urgent in both of our minds. And I realize how foolish it was to not have Taisa by my side, on my side, since the very beginning of my medical odyssey with CMV.

Not only is Taisa forthright and honest, but she's also probably the most high-energy person I know. We can barely go on walks together because I can't keep up with her long, unstoppable legs. Three months before I had Naomi, Taisa gave birth to her first baby, and she's already back at work full time, able to pump copious amounts of milk, and has somehow also had time to bake Christmas cookies, whip up borscht for us, and pick up lattes that she's brought over to my house. We're sitting on the couch, nursing our babies (which takes her a third of the time it takes me), when I tell her what's going on at Lutheran.

Without stopping to think about any pushback or what people at work will think of her, she says, "I'll email the right people at Lutheran about CMV. I'll do it today."

———

Taisa's email is professional and direct. She cc's me—which I so appreciate, rather than being left to wonder what was said between two doctors, as though I don't need to know—on her email to the infectious disease pharmacist at Lutheran. In the email, Taisa asks why there isn't a protocol for CMV testing at Lutheran. She mentions the new FDA-approved CMV saliva swab that could be used—and processed—at the hospital so parents don't have to wait for the baby to pee into a bag or wait days for results.

Taisa writes that coming up with a CMV testing protocol specific to Lutheran *is an interim fix because there's an application to put CMV on the RUSP,* which is true. She's talking about the Recommended Uniform Screening Panel: a list of congenital diseases compiled by the federal government—a menu of sorts—from which each state can select the conditions to test for automatically, right after birth, using the newborn dried bloodspot. Two CMV mothers, on behalf of the National CMV Foundation, have just submitted a two-hundred-page request to include CMV on the RUSP, meaning we'd be one huge step closer to having *all* American newborns tested for CMV, as soon as they're born, through their blood—a model called "universal" testing.

Taisa knows what I told her over coffee: that even though congenital CMV isn't on the RUSP, it's actually more common than thirty-four of the thirty-six core conditions on the RUSP put together. A big reason CMV isn't on the RUSP is that the medical committee that created the RUSP for the federal government over a decade ago, in 2004, had little experience in infectious diseases, so they "deferred decision-making" on CMV until a later date. And the National CMV Foundation's submission to add CMV to the RUSP won't be processed for another three to five years.

For now, should Lutheran agree to do so, it will be able to accommodate only "targeted" testing for CMV—that is, testing only the babies who fail their hearing tests—and this will be accomplished through a urine catch or a saliva swab. It's Taisa's last sentence about the hospital's failure to acknowledge CMV at all in newborns that moves me to tears: *I love our hospital, but clearly this is a huge lapse in what should be the standard of care.*

———

The pharmacist is awesome. She's pragmatic and direct. She writes back: *Do you think the conditional approach is going to remain the standard? I just have a hard time understanding why we wouldn't just screen every baby.*

If only the entire medical system could see things so clearly. If only this were the guiding principle in our approach to taking care of CMV. It will take me some time to figure out why testing every baby at every hospital isn't quite as simple as it seems.

For now, I email the Lutheran team—which seems to be growing—my humble opinion that targeted testing should be the first step but not the last. Because it isn't enough. I attach a study from the Alabama epidemiologist Dr. Karen Fowler, who insists that using a "targeted" testing model means we'll still miss an unacceptable number of newborns infected with CMV: 43 percent, to be exact.

Because, remember, CMV is usually asymptomatic at birth. That means the newborns who pass their hearing tests, who look healthy in their mothers' arms, who are silently harboring CMV, will go home from the hospital, and their parents will probably never hear of CMV for the rest of that child's life—even if the child ends up with deafness, blindness, or cognitive delays.

Children who are asymptomatic at birth do tend to be much less affected than those born with symptoms. But years later a French doctor I meet at the International CMV Conference in Alabama will tell me she's never seen a true lifelong "asymptomatic" case; all these children have behavioral or health issues that haven't been attributed to their diagnoses with congenital CMV.

Universal testing is obviously important for identifying more children at risk of lifelong complications from CMV. But maybe less obviously, it's also critical that we test *all* babies because administering the test wouldn't be education- or income-dependent; it wouldn't require a child's parents to ask for the test and pay for it. Universal testing would be a step in the direction of health equity. And studies estimate it would be cost-effective for the healthcare system, too.

Until then, we're not just lacking data on how many children with CMV have symptoms of it; we're also lacking knowledge of what's called the "cumulative disease burden" of the disease—how many kids truly have it, and how much it is costing insurers and the medical system and CMV parents and our kids.

The Lutheran pharmacist is with me; she's in favor of eventual universal testing. But she reveals another aspect of the medical hesitancy to address CMV when she writes back to me: *Historically speaking, physicians, medical directors, etc., don't like to be the "first" to do anything.*

4

I like to be the first. I like to compete in races, start programs in schools and hospitals that don't have them, send out the first invitation. A lot of times this ends in failure or embarrassment, but it's better than wondering what I could have changed.

That winter, as we're going about our lives at Zaley's school, at church, at the Deaf school program, I realize that all our communities have *place,* this thing that I know is important because it has so long complicated my life. It strikes me that I need to meet some of these CMV mothers in person, stand in a kitchen, admire our children—and that I will take the lead.

When I post on the CMV Mommies page to see how many mothers live in Colorado and want to meet at my house, only seven moms respond. But it's a start.

Because it's the holidays and flu season, five people end up bailing the day of the CMV gathering. Anna and Zaley wake up mildly sick. But I can't cancel after how much the two remaining moms have expressed they want to come, how much they've shifted other obligations to attend. A few hours before everyone is coming over, Luke takes the girls down to his parents', and I stay home, cleaning the house while Naomi naps, setting out wineglasses, and arranging a ring of Ritz crackers and slices of elk summer sausage on a plate.

The doorbell rings and I open it to see Richelle—a no-nonsense mother of five who drove all the way down from the farm town of Greeley and who's wearing Carhartts and a loose hoodie and carrying a cheesecake. Her daughter Sami is eight and in hospice; she couldn't come because it's winter and too risky with germs. (Sami wears a vest twice a day that rattles her body rapidly, so she won't choke on the fluids in her lungs.) A few minutes later the doorbell rings again, and it's a woman who looks like Richelle's polar opposite. Ashley is a young single mom from Colorado Springs who's wearing heavy eye makeup, a lacy shirt, and heels. Her daughter with CMV, Avalee, didn't come either because of the long drive. Avalee is ten and has autism, hearing loss, and cerebral palsy due to CMV. Both women have driven at least ninety minutes to get here, and outside, it has started snowing.

We fill plates with food that was intended for ten. We settle in the family room and start with stories about each of our kids. We talk about how our kids with CMV are doing. We talk about how we're doing ourselves. Ashley can barely keep it together some weeks, she says, with two girls and all the therapies and no father figure to help. (Ashley is also a Special Olympics coach, works full time, and will soon win Colorado Mother of the Year.) Richelle says that as much as she's imagined Sami's last days, it's becoming more and more difficult as the family actually approaches them. Sami was recently hospitalized and Richelle wasn't sure she'd ever come back home.

Richelle also has a different take on CMV than I've ever heard.

Richelle's husband had a vasectomy after their first four children. Eight years later Richelle found out she was pregnant with Sami. "It was medically impossible," she says, remembering they'd gone back to the urologist to have her husband checked, to see if there'd been a small loophole where his sperm had swum through. "The surgery had been done flawlessly, and the doctor said there was literally no way my husband had gotten me pregnant."

The doctor then fixed Richelle with his eyes like this might be the time to admit to an extramarital affair.

"Of course it was my husband who got me pregnant with Sami!" she says, throwing her arms up and laughing. "But it was a miracle. That's why we've always accepted CMV. Sami was never even supposed to happen. CMV was part of her from the very beginning, and we believe CMV is the reason we had her."

This is different than what I've heard before: *We were given this child with CMV for a reason.* Richelle seems to be saying the opposite:

CMV was the reason.

———

About half an hour after the women arrive, there's a huge crash in our basement, like someone has come in through a window and is going to hold us all hostage. My instinct is to call 911. Or run. The three of us are sitting in the family room, wide-eyed, looking at each other and waiting for someone to move.

"What should we do?" I ask these women who've basically just arrived.

"Let's go see!" Richelle says, shooting up from the couch without skipping a beat. She pulls her pants up by the waist and marches straight into the kitchen. I point toward the basement, and she follows my finger without hesitation. In my head, she's about to be dragged back up the stairs, at knifepoint, and into the yard. My heart is pounding in my chest as we descend behind her into the darkness because the light switch for our basement is, senselessly, at the bottom of the stairs. I click it on.

When we round the corner, I see immediately what had happened: a Pack 'n' Play has crashed to the ground from where either Luke or I had balanced it on a tower of totes, knocking down all the totes as it fell, and spilling their contents all over the floor.

When we go back upstairs and sit down, laughing and sighing with relief, Ashley says one night someone broke into her house while she and her two girls were upstairs, sleeping. The burglars had taken electronics and jewelry before she woke up in the morning. She still lives there. It had scared the shit out of her, but what was she supposed to do?

"I'm the mother of my children," she says. "My only purpose is to protect them."

———

At the end of the night, while we're standing in the kitchen and swiping the last ribbons of chocolate off the cheesecake platter, Ashley puts her hands in her pockets and says, with tears in her eyes, "I've been looking for you guys for a long, long time." We say goodbye, and I tell them I hope I'll get to meet their girls sometime soon.

But I never do meet Sami. She will die the following February, on Richelle's birthday. I will always regret that I missed the chance to meet her.

When they leave, I write everything down. I have come to accept that there are seasons for everything: seasons for writing, seasons for nursing, seasons for reading, seasons for sleep training (which obliterates all other seasons).

Some people insist that to be a writer, you must not make it seasonal: you must sit down and write every day. I reject this idea. Because writing with young kids can look like a paragraph a week. Sometimes it can look like not writing for a month. Sometimes, when the muse visits, when it just randomly works, I sit up in bed and write ten thousand words in one night. Newly motivated by Ashley and Richelle, I put the finishing touches on my email to the agent in New York and hit send.

The rest of that winter is mild, with snow like it falls in Sitka, gently decorating the tallest of trees. Zaley starts reading. Anna starts saying short sentences: "Lovey you." "Where Zayyyy-eee?" And Naomi is so predictable as to seem formulaic. She wakes, she eats, she sleeps, and most amazingly, she *stays* asleep. (Anna won't sleep through the night for nearly three years.) This baby is so easy, we decide we'll go on a trip.

It's late February—Naomi is three months old, Anna is two and a half, and Zaley is five—when we book tickets to Arizona with Luke's whole side of the family. Seventeen of us will be staying on the outskirts of Phoenix at a modest resort with a lazy river, a water slide, and multiple pools.

Despite the particular hell of travel with young kids, I'm excited to go. I love cacti, outdoor swimming, and the desert's dry hues. Plus, I have an ulterior motive: Kathleen Muldoon lives in Phoenix. At the end of our stay, I've arranged to meet Kathleen and Gideon, her son.

Even though I've been dreaming of a poolside vacation since my children were born, once we arrive in Phoenix, I know it will be different than I'd imagined. While the other kids Anna's age are running around the resort confidently and looking over their shoulders as their moms call to them, I have to restrict all of Anna's movements with either my arms or my signing hands.

Luke and I have continued to learn ASL on a weekly basis, with Lori—and now our new teacher Cathy, whom we love equally—but our desire to use two languages hasn't been adopted by our kids. I don't realize till it's too late that we should have practiced more ASL with Anna before our trip. Anna doesn't understand sentences of sign language, just single words and phrases from children's books that lack context at the pool (*spaghetti, ditch, I like myself*). She seems bothered by sign language here, moving her head to the side to see around my moving hands when I sign. And for the first time ever, she doesn't want to wear her cochlear implants.

I've brought longer-lasting lithium batteries than her normal ones. But every time I put the implants on her head, in their waterproof sleeves, they turn orange, and she slaps them off her scalp.

I won't find out till we're home and I'm talking to our audiologist, Allison, that lithium batteries don't work in airtight waterproof sleeves. Lithium needs oxygen to work.

———

The first few days of the trip to Arizona, I'm testy and self-centered. It's not that I want Anna to be like all the other kids, but I do want to enjoy vacation like all the other mothers. And besides not wearing her implants, Anna keeps falling over. Her Achilles tendons still angle inward, and because her braces would be cumbersome at the pool (necessitating socks and shoes), she isn't wearing them. Every time she falls, she gets right back up and tries again to walk—right alongside a very deep pool. This perseverance will serve her well in the future, but it serves *me* poorly right now.

Everyone is so helpful. Luke's dad bounces Naomi to sleep around the perimeter of the pool. Luke teaches Zaley to swim, fetches me snacks, directs Max and his other young brother, Jude, to the next of our needs. But all Anna wants to do is sit in the hot tub, which is removed from the rest of the family by a flight of stairs and a giant rock wall. I don't blame her. This is the best way to take care of a body: give it water, warmth, rest, and stillness. It's a remedy less profound-seeming than many, but important nonetheless—when the physical body is tended to, so are illnesses, sorrow, and malcontent.

Yup'ik people know this. That's why Father and his kids are hammering together a wooden hut in their front yard, where a fifty-five-gallon drum will become a woodstove, and water poured over scalding rocks will steam the space up to two hundred degrees. The *maqivik* was also where midwives were traditionally trained in how to deliver babies, where diseases were expelled, where the mourners of the dead gathered to grieve. Similar to a Russian *banya*—or a hot tub at a resort in Arizona—it's a place where you alternate silence with storytelling, where you see how much the body can endure.

The hot tub is where I spend most of the vacation when I'm not nursing the baby. It's too hot for some kids, but Anna loves it. When people ask her name and how old she is, she stares back at them, deaf, glassy-eyed, and completely content.

5

When Friday arrives, I'm excited. I don't have to pull on a damp, cold swimsuit and find all the girls' accessories for the pool. I'm going to meet Gideon and Kathleen. While Luke lathers the kids' soft arms with sunscreen, finds goggles, and gathers a pile of somewhat dry towels, I shower, dry my hair, and find a notebook and a pen. I love feeling like a writer alongside being a mother. Sometimes I wish being one didn't mean leaving behind the other, but that's what it requires. Sometimes I'm not sure why I keep expecting things to be easy, when nothing ever is.

I'm also a little nervous. I want to do Kathleen and Gideon's story the justice it deserves—to voice, on their behalf, the details that CMV has historically been denied.

When I get in the rental car and put the address into my phone, I'm surprised and relieved: Gideon's school, the Foundation for Blind Children, is seven blocks from our hotel. I could have walked. I drive because I'm late. I pass by strip malls and Checks Cashed stores, halfway hoping I've entered the wrong address. Then I see it: the school appears out of nowhere, like a circular spaceship set down where it wasn't supposed to land.

The architecture is pristine and dramatic, with spherical windows randomly scattered around a beige, stucco-like base. I will later learn that these small, round windows were designed to prevent light from flooding in and changing throughout the day—it's easier for blind children to learn in level, consistent light. The roofline echoes the surrounding mountains, jutting up in triangular protrusions of copper. In fact, the roof design pays homage to the accomplishment of the CEO's thirteen-year-old son: he was the youngest blind person to summit the peak of Mount Kilimanjaro, in 2009, with a group of other blind children from the school.

The thoughtfulness of the building makes me think immediately of the Rocky Mountain Deaf School in Denver—the vibrant colors, the sprawling care taken with every inch of the school, the same care-taking that I have to assume extends to the staff and students inside. Inside, a green metal wall with no seams in its surface (so students trailing their hands won't catch them) runs from one end of the open front office to the other, and like all the other architectural details, its design reflects the achievements of the blind: this one signifies the 1.5-mile swim to Alcatraz that a group of students from the school completed.

These feats are all impressive, and yet they sadden me too: I know they're things the boy I'm about to meet may never be able to do. I'm not sure if this is an honest way to feel or an ableist way to frame his life.

I haven't yet met a child with CMV—or any disease, actually—as severely affected as Gideon. I arrive before Kathleen and stand in the waiting room as elementary-age and older blind children come in the glass doors with their caregivers. Some have walking sticks, others are led by a loving arm. Some wear glasses, others have eyes that don't open. I speak with the director about their teen-to-work program, wondering if Gideon will ever have a job.

Then I see Gideon and Kathleen coming toward the door. Kathleen is carrying her son, and an older woman is with them, pushing a small, stroller-like wheelchair up to the sliding-glass doors. When they come in the entryway, I introduce myself, and Kathleen introduces her mom, who's in town from Canada for the week. I step to Kathleen's side so I can see Gideon's face. He's snuggled against his mother's chest, and one bright eye is peering out at me from behind royal blue glasses. I've seen handfuls of pictures of this child online, and yet in person, he's different than I expected.

He's much smaller than he looks in pictures. And his hair is even more luscious—his thick brown waves looks like they'll spring back up if you push them down, which I kind of want to do. His smile seems distinctly intended for me. When I touch his arm and ask, "How's your morning?" his eyes go upward in pleasure, and his open smile grows by a centimeter on each side.

Kathleen tells me we'll be in the gymnasium, where there's a Friday-morning program for preschoolers. In the bright, expansive gym, a woman is reading a book on a mat, and an interpreter is signing next to her. "A lot of these kids are visually impaired but very visually motivated," Kathleen, leaning over to me, explains.

Most of the kids are sitting on mats with their mothers, a striking number of whom look young—in their twenties. They're swaying with their toddlers, stroking their hair, bringing their small hands up to feel the faces of their caregivers. Whereas a room full of typical kids might contain mothers on their phones, these mothers seem intently focused on their young. They are touching them at all times, on various points, cueing them to sounds, signs, light, and touch.

In a corner where we can quietly talk to each other, Kathleen pours a thick, raspberry-colored smoothie into a bottle while Gideon gazes up from her lap. He groans with anticipation of his breakfast, starting to squirm as she finishes pouring it from one container to another. Then she puts the bottle to his lips, and he sucks. I'm impressed he's eating solid foods.

"He's on a blended diet," she explains. "He has a G-tube, but he also loves to eat. I make huge batches of these and freeze them in one-ounce ice cube trays. This one has blueberries, avocado, coconut oil, almonds, and beets."

I know Kathleen still works full time as a professor and has two other children to take care of—one older than Gideon, and one younger. I remember another CMV mother online saying that having a child severely disabled by CMV is like having a newborn all the time. And yet Kathleen seems to handle Gideon's needs with aplomb and with love. I ask her how she balances his needs with the needs of her other children—an issue I'm struggling with at home. "It's a high priority that all my kids feel they get attention," she responds. "But they also understand the structure of our lives. From the beginning, we've always made clear that we need to pay close attention to Gideon and what he needs."

Then I ask her to tell me about the beginning—when she first found out he had CMV.

"The pediatrician was washing his hands," Kathleen remembers of that day. "And he wouldn't turn to look at us. 'I don't know how to tell you this,' he said, 'but I think it's congenital CMV.'"

"It was like a crack in the planet," she tells me. "Seth collapsed in a chair. They loaded Gideon into a glass case, and then they took him away."

Gideon did take valganciclovir, which could be why he still has some of his hearing. Though Kathleen will never know exactly when she contracted CMV, often babies impacted during the first trimester have outcomes like Gideon. He has the type of vision impairment that means his brain doesn't make meaning of sight. He can see stairs, for example, but not understand that they lead up or down.

When I ask Kathleen if there's anything she would change about Gideon if she could, she tells me, "I have no sympathy for my life." I have seen evidence of this, and it's totally true. Online, if you're friends with Kathleen, you know that she's very realistic about Gideon's challenges and also very clear about her family's sense of joy. She makes their Halloween costumes every year, and they're downright amazing. In one photo, Gideon is wearing a Superman costume with a cape, and his wheelchair is encased in a painted box. The box depicts a city skyline at night, and on the back half of it, perfectly lined up with Gideon's upper body, are stuffed legs in Superman's tights, making it appear that Gideon's legs are behind him, his body a superhero's in flight.

Gideon absolutely loves music—Yo-Yo Ma, sometimes Punch Brothers, and always Andrew Bird. He also loves school, and when I ask if he's always as happy as he is right now, Kathleen says, "Yes, he really is. He's a super social, happy kid."

Gideon uses an adaptive communication device that's controlled by his eyes. When they linger on the image of a word for more than a half second, that means he's making a deliberate choice in what to say. By second grade, Gideon will communicate in sentences, divulge secrets to his mom, and understand chapter books like *Stink,* which his mom and dad read to him aloud. Their goal is for him to be in a mainstream classroom by fifth grade, with a one-on-one teacher who works with the deafblind. I realize now that any assumption I'd had about Gideon likely isn't true. But I ask Kathleen how she fights for an end to CMV while also saying Gideon is worth having.

"It's too big of a problem for me to teach everyone that all life has value," Kathleen says. "What I can do is take my kid to Target with us when we go and show everyone the fun we're having and allow him access to his voice so he can share himself with the world. People will see that it's not scary to be different, and the more we talk about it, the more normalized it becomes."

———

After the storytime part of the program, there's free play, during which some of the mobile kids bounce huge balls around the room with their teachers and OTs. Kathleen places Gideon under a home-made activity mat—a PVC pipe on two vertical PVC stands. The horizontal pipe is strung with bright ribbons and star-spangled tinsel. Bells, too, dangle down, which a child could grab if they had use of their hands, and which we jangle for Gideon, who laughs and lolls his head from side to side.

Gideon lost all his hearing in one ear in the last six months, and I understand that their journey toward cochlear implants will be much different than it was with Anna for us. For one, Gideon has been hearing his whole life, so to call it hearing *loss* is much more fitting in their situation than ours. Kathleen articulates the other difference between our situations when she says, "When we first found out he had CMV, Seth and I just kept saying to each other, 'Maybe he'll only be deaf.'"

I swallow, digesting that my initial grief with Anna, though huge-feeling at the time, had been so much smaller than what Kathleen's family had experienced and would continue to experience with their son. One of the greatest lessons CMV has imparted to me is relativity: that you don't really know where you are in your struggles until you know other people and theirs.

This is not to say that suffering should be contested or compared. There is no answering to the discrepancies of suffering, no score-board, no adjusting we can make. I think of what Father Gnocchi wrote, about the mysterious social economy we share, which doses out health, wealth, tragedy, and death, and though we don't second-guess our inheritance of the positive aspects of life, so many of us fail to understand why we might suffer as well.

Gnocchi does not offer the exact *why* of suffering, but he does suggest its effects: "The loving and unexhausted efforts of science; the many different works of human solidarity; the marvels of supernatural charity."

I see all of these so clearly in Kathleen.

———

Despite Kathleen's self-professed, generally happy demeanor—one she has likely passed down to her son—the tears still come. "One of the hardest things," Kathleen says, wiping her eyes and smiling at Gideon under his stars, "is the nights when I lie awake, wondering if he will die, or if I will first. Or if, before that, he'll be sexually assaulted, which is statistically much more likely to happen than not."

She explains that people who are deaf, blind, or have issues with their mobility are victimized by crime at a higher rate than the rest of the population. In fact, children like Gideon with developmental or intellectual delays are four to ten times more likely to be sexually abused —a statistic that makes me queasy with fury.

Kathleen and Seth's overarching priority for Gideon is communication—to give him a voice. "Our number-one thing," she says, "is that we make sure he comes out of school with an understanding that his words have meaning. And," she adds, "to wait his turn." Kathleen and I both laugh that Gideon has this same problem that all kids share. But she explains: "This school only goes to fourth grade. So when he goes back to the district school, they can take away his communication device if he's speaking out of turn. This would be the worst kind of punishment. We need him to be patient so he can be a reliable reporter, so he can be understood."

———

I do wonder what Kathleen thinks of me being there—what she thinks of my *New York Times* piece that has just come out about our experience with CMV. For Gideon, there's always the next-appearing thing: an illness he can't handle, another diagnosis (he will need a massive hip surgery in a matter of years), further hearing loss, the looming complications of any hospital stay.

When I ask this of Kathleen—how do I have a right to tell the story of CMV?—she refutes my self-consciousness immediately. "Your pain, your journey, your joy, are absolutely yours. Everyone has a story no matter what."

She also feels that in order to get people to care about CMV and our kids, we need to show the world the whole spectrum. Then she tells me something I didn't know before. After her TORCH test, she Googled CMV, and upon seeing a child severely disabled by CMV, she shook it off, assuring herself that wouldn't happen to them. She believes that showing an audience only the children most affected by CMV would drive fear, not positive change.

She also points out that while she can control Gideon's world, she'd be terrified to have a child like Anna who may be less protected by nature of her being mobile. Anna will have to figure out her differences, on her own, in a discriminatory world.

"The thing that you have is the thing that you learn to manage," Kathleen says. "Anything else can seem too hard to bear."

———

I think again of the warrior beads and how many Gideon might have on his necklace. Then I think of the string holding the beads together. What does that represent? No one had said. But then, looking at Gideon, I realize the simple answer: the through line of a medically complicated child's struggles is their life itself—something that can't be qualified or quantified, as much as we always want to inquire about how chronically ill children are doing (not super great, usually), or how long they'll live (no one knows).

In fact, one CMV mom online posted: *People ask me all the time, "How long does he have to live?"* Her response: *What, do you think he has an expiration date printed on his ass??*

As if Kathleen knows what I'm thinking, she points to a child with trisomy 13 who's playing with his mother a few feet away. "It can be hard to see past the body," she says. "But no one should presume what a child can do. That child wasn't even supposed to live a year."

The boy's teeth are triangular, his eyes only white behind tightly drawn lids. His mother plays with him as any mother might play with her three-year-old boy. Or maybe not, maybe I see something deeper between them, as he holds stackable cups and maneuvers them. I think then of something Kathleen wrote online about Gideon: *My son is beloved and whole and human and amazing.*

———

After I say goodbye to Gideon and Kathleen, I walk to the front of the school and realize that I don't want to leave. I want to spend all day here, and I'm hesitant to return to the hotel, where I'll inevitably try to articulate the differences between Gideon and Anna. I fear the prejudices of my own language. And I don't want to drive back to the pettiness of my problems—the distance of the hot tub from the pool, the cochlear implant malfunctions, the menial frustrations of languages that are "no-tech," as Kathleen calls Gideon's ways of saying yes and no without a device. (Yes is looking up, and no is tilting his head to the right.)

I drive away from Phoenix for a few minutes and toward a mountain trail called Dreamy Draw, where we'd hiked a few days before. As I walk into the desert, my mind reaches for reason, for an explanation of illness among people of such goodness. On a high, steep ledge, I look out over the land, where both the exquisiteness of the desert and the ruin of the city are stretched out before me. This is how it is: a landscape of pain, a landscape of beauty, all of it inexplicable, ongoing.

———

That afternoon, back at the poolside, I stare. I watch all the people go about their usual things: they walk and run and swim and trot up steps and shriek down the slide. They call to each other, turn, listen, laugh, respond. They spread sunscreen, eat nachos, pack bags, slip on their flip-flops. People gripe about the clouds, the wet towels, the prices, the water temperature. They snuggle sitting babies, drift on inner tubes, pile hair in ponytails, sip piña coladas through hot pink straws. It is all so wonderful, everything everyone is doing, and they are all so able-bodied and able to understand, and no one even knows it. Kathleen once wrote that her family experiences "the million paper cuts of everyday ableism," and I wonder if so many of those cuts are simply our obliviousness, how we mistake any life, mobile or not, for anything short of miraculous.

I want to stand at the top of the water slide and call down to them, *Look at all this you have, all this you can do,* but it would be futile and crazy, and then I realize something is missing. It's Gideon. It isn't just Gideon himself, it's the way he'd changed everything I can see. I want for everyone everywhere to know someone like him. How differently we might live.

I am quieter on a lawn chair than I usually am. I sign *Hot water?* To Anna, and she nods her fist and, with no volume control, yells YES!

The hot tub is full of mellow strangers. Anna's body floats back against mine, finding the same place where she started—at first, a gathering of cells, then blood and lungs, heart and head, heels and ears. She is so silent and so light of weight, as she was in the beginning, before her name, before we knew she was anything other than herself.

We float and we breathe. Across the scrim of heat, I see something. Two adult sisters—one Deaf and one hearing, I'll find out. They are signing to each other in the steam.

6

Erin, the lawyer, is so organized, I feel like a bad person. We are meeting with a Colorado state senator named Cheri Jahn, and prior to this introduction, Erin has compiled a binder with both of our families' stories and general information about CMV. When I meet her at a Starbucks in Arvada, Erin's straight blond hair and shiny ironed clothes are impeccable, as though she's already won a trial before I had time to shower. Her husband, Jeff, is sitting at a table with her, plus their neighbor John, who's a lobbyist, and we chat with four thick binders before us, waiting for the senator to walk in. Senator Jahn has already received a copy of everything by email, Erin says. "I just hope she read it!" she admits—laughing fast, then stopping fast, too. We're all a little on edge that the senator won't take up our cause.

When Senator Jahn enters the coffee shop, she exudes officiality. She's in her sixties, wearing a velvet blazer, a long velvet scarf, and heels. She spots us and says she'll be right over. She seems rushed. She orders her coffee, then plops down at the table. She pulls off her scarf, places both hands on the dark wooden surface, and says, "So. Tell me about this CMV."

Erin and I exchange glances. We will, despite Erin's hours of preparation, have to start at the beginning. But the senator is attentive and sharp, asking questions about incidence rates in our state, treatments for newborns, how Matthew and Anna are doing. Erin answers all her questions with professionalism and insight. She also reveals that Matthew is showing early signs of autism.

Then the senator asks the big one: "What about testing during pregnancy?"

Doctors in many European countries (France, Belgium, Spain, Italy, Germany, Austria, Portugal, Israel, and the Netherlands, specifically) do routinely test pregnant women for CMV, but I tell the senator that we do not here.

While it's true that routine testing during pregnancy would likely drive awareness, if you ask me, most OBs in the United States aren't yet educated enough about CMV for regular testing during pregnancy to be worth the confusion and risk.

The situation goes like this: When friends of mine have requested CMV antibody tests from their OBs, almost all of them have received serious pushback and the sentiment from their doctors that they needn't worry about CMV. Some are convinced by this and come back to me with skepticism, wondering if CMV is actually too rare for their effort or attention. But if a friend persists and gets the test, her OB usually doesn't counsel her appropriately about the results. They'll either send her into a panic if she has short-term antibodies—which could very well be false, as short-term antibodies have a high false positive rate, tell her that she has antibodies to CMV, therefore she doesn't need to worry about it—which, again, isn't true because you can always be reinfected by a new strain; or email her antibody values that are indecipherable to a lay person and never explaining their import. One friend of mine who was pregnant with her fourth and had three very young kids ended up having no antibodies to CMV, and her OB did not counsel her about her elevated risk. He said to her: "Don't worry, CMV is only really an issue in hospitals, not in preschool settings."

I stopped recommending that pregnant friends get tested for CMV unless they see, on ultrasound, the following things: echogenic bowel, hydrops, placental enlargement, intrauterine growth restriction, enlarged liver or spleen, or microcephaly (which Anna exhibited on a scan at thirty-six weeks, to which my OB had remarked, "We'll just have to wait and see.") A pregnant woman should also be tested for CMV if she's experiencing a mono-like illness. And she should be tested, without condescension, if she simply wants the test.

But after that, the doctor's correct interpretation of data and delivery of that knowledge is critical.

Wondering why this humane conversation about CMV seems to be such a rarity in the United States, I once pressed an Italian friend of mine who moved to Sitka why she thought women were so readily tested and informed in Italy, where there's universal health coverage, largely free of charge. "Doctors take their responsibility differently in Italy," she told me. "They take it seriously that their role is to *serve*."

She may be right. And jamming the American healthcare system with millions of CMV tests that aren't well explained could cause unintended outcomes at both ends of the pregnancy spectrum: on the one end, more panic; on the other end, more false security.

"I think instead of screening for CMV during pregnancy," Dr. Boppana told me, "the most appropriate practice should be to counsel all pregnant women about CMV and congenital CMV and the exposures and behaviors that increase the risk."

The Society for Maternal-Fetal Medicine agrees. Silence is not a healthy or ethical way to handle the reality of CMV.

———

The senator is nodding after I tell her we're focusing on testing babies right after birth, since testing during pregnancy is more complicated. She is retiring at the end of this term, she says, but she thinks she can "push something through." She thinks our best bet is to go for the low-hanging fruit: add a CMV education amendment to an existing bill that's about to be heard on the floor.

That bill is Colorado's Infant Newborn Screening Act, which seeks to update the DBS (the Newborn Dried Blood Spot test) and the newborn hearing test programs in Colorado. The legislation for Colorado's newborn screenings hasn't been updated in twenty years, and it lacks clear authority for who follows up with babies' families when they're diagnosed with hearing loss or congenital disease.

I know that babies who are "lost to follow-up" are at risk for lifelong language and developmental delays. And I know this could have been us.

———

Our first official meeting to discuss the CMV amendment is at the state capitol, where I haven't been since elementary school. Luke is at home with our kids, Erin and Jeff are already inside the stately building, and I can't find a place to park.

Once I do, I'm ten minutes late, and I trot inside, where men and women in pressed suits are rushing between rooms. I feel both purposeful and small. I'm here for a reason, but I don't know where to go. I move to the center of the building and look up briefly at the soaring, golden rotunda. I remember standing here as a girl, in fourth grade, knowing I didn't want to be a legislator but a writer, and feeling intimidated by the outward display of importance in places like this.

"Megan!" I hear Erin calling. She and Jeff are standing near the door to the offices of the Colorado Department of Public Health and Environment (CDPHE). I follow them inside.

The official who welcomes us into the meeting room is a guy with dark gelled hair who's very thin and very young. Like, possibly fresh out of college. I get the sense, immediately, that he's there because this meeting is on his agenda, not because it interests him. "We can't really add anything to the bill," he says before we've even sat down. "But we understand that you want to talk about CMV, and we understand your concerns."

He has that predictable, disingenuous-sounding cadence of speech common to corporations and large organizations. I distrust him immediately. There's also a middle-aged man in the room who has stood up from the table to shake our hands, and he seems warmer, maybe more patient. John, the lobbyist, takes out copies of our amendment and places them before everyone. Erin and I have already seen this language multiple times; we've been revising it along with the senator and a few doctors from the local chapter of the American Academy of Pediatrics. Our red lines appear on the document, asking the state to take more responsibility than we know they will.

We flip through this document for a few minutes, seeing where CDPHE has struck things out. Erin and I urge the officials to eventually consider a program like they have in Utah, where the department of health directs a public education program to inform all women about CMV. In Utah, CMV messaging appears on buses and billboards and in public service announcements on TV. A CMV mom named Sarah Doutré was largely responsible for this legislation authorizing the program—the first such legislation in any state. Sarah's daughter Daisy was identified with CMV at fifteen months, when she lost her hearing completely. It helped that Daisy's grandmother, Ronda, was a Utah state senator. It also helped that they secured ongoing funding for CMV awareness and change—$70,000 a year from the legislature, allocated to the Utah Department of Health.

The Colorado officials, on the other hand, are not open to the idea of a program that would place any fiscal responsibility on them. They ask us if we plan to raise that money ourselves.

There's a projector in the room, and the younger of the two officials turns it on. "We wanted to show you that we worked with another CMV mom some years ago to publicize CMV around town."

I'm taken aback when Karina and Jayden appear on the screen, featured in a brochure I've never seen. It's blue and green, and while I love the pictures, it doesn't look professionally designed. But I'm hopeful, for an instant, that this agency does want to listen, that they might be swayed to change the impact of CMV in our state. The older public health employee is talking about how they placed this flyer at various locations around Denver and did their part to make it visible, as evidenced by the CDPHE logo in the corner of the page.

"Can I ask a question?" I say. "Where exactly did you put this flyer? I've never seen it anywhere in person or online."

Both of the officials think for a moment. Then the older one says, "You know, I can't remember."

The younger official jumps in with an offer—one of the things we've already proposed in the amendment. "We are more than happy to create a page on our website devoted to congenital CMV."

I think about something that somehow hadn't really occurred to me in the editing of the amendment. When I'd been in the hospital after giving birth to Anna; when I'd feared her smallness and silence; when the doctors had cycled in and out; when I'd needed to figure out nursing; when I'd needed to care for the wounds of my own body; when I was as tired as a newborn myself—would I ever have gotten out my phone, gone to the CDPHE website, and found a link to CMV—a link that, to this day, still doesn't show up when you go to their "Diseases A to Z" page?

Two years ago I might have been less assertive, might have accepted this meager offer from a state agency whose mission states that it "continues to identify and respond to emerging issues affecting Colorado's public and environmental health." But not today. I'm tired of health-based mission statements. I'm tired of reading them for their irony. And I know too much about CMV to politely accept a useless shred of acknowledgement without pointing out how pointless it is.

"I know this is what we agreed upon in our emails," I say. "But let's be honest. This information will never make its way into the hands of a woman who's just had a baby."

"Well," the young one says. "For now, that's the best we can do."

———

When a group of CMV mothers are asked to convene at the capitol with our children to support the amendment, I put Anna in a pair of black tights and her favorite silver-threaded sweater dress. I pull her hair up into a ponytail, so that people can see her cochlear implants, which sport new leopard-print decals that she picked out herself.

When we arrive at the capitol, I hold Anna and carry her halfway up the circular stairs I climbed as a child. When we stop, I take her chin between my finger and thumb and direct her eyes up to the latticework of the stunning dome. I tell her, with tears in my eyes, that this time, being here is way more special than any other time I've been: we are here because of her.

Upstairs, in an atrium where we will wait more than four hours to be heard, the other children with CMV are a perfect representation of its spectrum: Ashley is there with Avalee, who's talkative and high energy and uses a bright pink wheelchair. A mom named Kimberly is there with her daughter, Kelleigh, who doesn't use verbal language and has a tracheotomy. Erin's son Matthew is there too, and he steals the show, zooming around the shiny tile floors with his new titanium alloy walker on wheels. We wait and wait for our turn (something we're all accustomed to doing in the CMV community), but by the time Erin testifies on the amendment, Anna and I have already left to pick up Zaley from school.

———

Ultimately, the bill passes, which should feel like a triumph. But when Colorado's modernized Infant Newborn Screening program goes into effect, the operation essentially fails. The CDPHE posts information about it on their website but does not proactively share it with hospitals, and the complicated new database to record newborn screenings online won't be ready till 2020.

The CDPHE webpage on congenital CMV fails, too: the language makes no mention of toddlers in the list of ways you can contract the disease.

The other part of the bill—for the CDPHE to assist hospitals in disseminating information about CMV—is written carefully enough to not obligate them to do anything. I have never seen the public health department actively involved in any CMV change in Colorado.

I realize that CMV change will have to happen the other way: with mothers at the helm, effecting change pregnancy by pregnancy, baby by baby, story by story.

7

I've always wondered how doctors who've given birth to babies with CMV feel about the disease. Soon after our amendment passes in Colorado, I find out.

In Michigan, a baby girl named Odessa is born to two physicians, Megan Pesch and her husband, Tom. Odessa is their third child, born very close in age to their other girls, who are nineteen months and three years old. Tom's an internal medicine primary care doctor, and Megan is a developmental pediatrician. Megan's job is guiding families through childhood developmental disabilities—things like hearing loss, developmental delays, and autism.

When I call Megan, I ask her what I always ask CMV moms: to tell me about her pregnancy. Megan's was unremarkable and concluded with a fairly standard labor and delivery. When Odessa (which means "journey") was born, she seemed generally healthy, but she had petechiae and failed her hearing test. Megan thought, as I had with Anna, that Odessa would pass her hearing tests soon. Also, that the rash on her face was from being stuck briefly during labor, and all would be well.

At the hospital, no one tested Odessa for CMV. Ten weeks later, when Odessa had her two-hour auditory brainstem response test, her parents found out she was profoundly deaf.

Megan grieved hard. Then she did a bunch of genetic testing (which revealed nothing), requested that Odessa's urine be tested for CMV (which revealed she was, in fact, shedding CMV), and then set out to find Odessa's DBS—her newborn dried bloodspot.

But there's a problem with testing the DBS for CMV, Megan explains. If a state has saved a newborn's dried bloodspot specimen, you can extract DNA from one or more of the blood stamps and test it for a specific congenital disease—a laboratory test called a PCR assay. But when the PCR assay for CMV was assessed in the 1990s, it was only around 30 percent sensitive to detecting CMV in the bloodspot extraction.

This is why most infants are tested through their saliva or urine for congenital CMV. Saliva and urine assays are much more sensitive, detecting CMV accurately about 95 to 99 percent of the time.

But saliva and urine tests are problematic, too. They're expensive to implement. As opposed to the DBS—a specimen already obtained from every baby in every hospital—you have to put new programs in place to collect urine and saliva and test them for CMV, change the backend order in every computer system, and train nurses to capture fluids correctly.

And most important, if you want to test a baby for CMV after they're one month old, saliva and urine aren't an accurate indication of *congenital* disease. The baby may test positive for the kind of benign CMV they've contracted outside the womb, from a sibling, having lived in a household of others and their colds.

In the case of Odessa, she was ten weeks old when they found out she was deaf—too late for CMV in her urine to be conclusive. The DBS then, Megan explains, is a possible—though imperfect—option because some states retain the dried bloodspot cards in their banks for six months or longer. A child's heel-stamped card can reveal, in some cases, if CMV was in their system on day one.

When Megan requested Odessa's DBS, she was given outdated contact information from the infectious disease department and never got a response; the person she'd emailed had stopped working there five years before. Megan had to do the legwork herself to retrieve the card, then sent it across the country to be tested for CMV at the University of Washington.

The results came back: Odessa's newborn blood was positive for congenital CMV. Her head ultrasound then revealed calcifications and cysts, which can indicate a heightened risk of future seizures and developmental disabilities.

When Megan dug through her old notes from pediatric residency training, she was thinking the same thing all CMV moms think—*I should have known*—though as a doctor, she might have felt this to a more self-shaming degree: *How could I have forgotten?* The notes from a class she'd taken to prepare for the American Board of Pediatrics certifying exam answered that question.

The workshop had been a week-long, intensive review of general pediatric topics, including over four hours dedicated to infectious diseases. CMV had been covered on only two of the slides. Neither slide instructed these soon-to-be pediatricians on how to care for babies born with CMV. And prevention of CMV in pregnancy wasn't mentioned at all. She hadn't forgotten the details; she had never learned them.

"I didn't feel like I had a fighting chance," Megan says, thinking back on her pregnancy and not knowing about CMV, about how she kissed her toddler on the lips and finished waffles rejected by her preschooler. "I wish I could look back and be like, *I tried. I tried everything and this happened anyway.*"

Megan's story is important not just because she's a doctor admitting to the unethical absence of CMV in medicine, but also because Odessa, like Erin's son Matthew, will end up being diagnosed with autism—a condition often seen in children with congenital CMV. Research in the area is still emerging, but intrauterine infections and other conditions that can affect the placenta have long been thought to predispose a child to autism.

"Children with autism can struggle with social communication and certain restrictive or repetitive behaviors," Megan tells me. "It's like rolling a ball back and forth. When a child has autism, they might get excited to catch the ball, but then walk away with the ball. It may not be intuitive that they should then roll the ball back. But if you think about it with language, some kids don't come to it naturally that communication is a social interaction, a volleying back and forth. This sort of exchange is the foundation of communication in any form. Some kids need to be shown that there's value in that back and forth, and there's more to it than getting your own needs met."

This is a good metaphor for good medicine, I realize: it's about more than just getting individual needs met. It's about *communication*—

just as Kathleen said, just as Megan identifies as a core challenge of autism, just as I've known with Anna. And when communication works in medicine, we feel deeply known, partially healed, and we might end up trusting our doctors as much as ourselves.

I tell Megan I would have loved to have a doctor like her. A doctor who had a story that met mine. A doctor who valued exchange. A doctor who *knew*.

I enjoy talking to Megan because she doesn't sound like a doctor who's smarter than me (even though she is); she sounds like a person. She says a huge problem with CMV is that "we've done a shit job assessing all the burdens of the disease." We don't have accurate numbers on the correlation between CMV and autism, for instance, but it certainly exists. In a small Italian study conducted on newborn dried bloodspots, doctors found that the CMV infection rate in patients with autism was thirty times higher than in the general Italian population.

Megan is looking for these numbers in the United States. She and a doctor at the University of Minnesota named Mark Schleiss are on their way to recruiting four hundred children from Michigan with an existing diagnosis of autism. They're then testing these children's dried bloodspot cards for CMV. "It's tricky," says Megan, "because children with autism live very full lives—it's not like a disease that needs to be cured. It's another way of viewing the world and it's beautiful in many ways. I don't want to prevent or eliminate autism. But I do want to prevent babies from being infected by a virus that can invade their developing brains in utero, that can lead to severe or life-threatening conditions." She hopes that if a link between CMV and later autism risk is confirmed, early intervention could be put in place to support children and their families.

Megan says that even the most skeptical researchers she's worked with also happen to believe, in their hearts—like every CMV doctor I've personally spoken with—that *all* babies should be screened at birth for CMV. Megan finally illuminates for me why this isn't happening. "In order to achieve universal CMV testing, we need more data, and we need the right systems in place."

The most critical of these systems is a more sensitive DBS.

In 2021 a new study assessing the DBS will change everything.

———

Everywhere I go with Anna, I find age groups interested in congenital CMV. When she starts toddler gymnastics at the age of three, I tell the grandma sitting in the bleachers whose daughter is pregnant with her second child. I tell the kind high school student who's been assigned to help Anna one-on-one at the gym. And I talk about CMV with other parents at a place called Feel the Beat—a nonprofit dance studio for deaf and disabled children that has bone-conduction floors so the kids can feel sound through vibrational energy—and that opens, incredibly, a mile from our house.

But is there treatment? people always ask me, as though this is the only thing that justifies knowing about CMV. *Is there treatment for CMV during pregnancy?*

I don't believe this is the right question. I believe we've been conditioned to expect prescriptions instead of conversations in medicine. I believe the question should be *What can I do about CMV during pregnancy?*

The first answer is that knowledge itself is treatment.

And then if you're wanting to know about medication, the tentative answer is yes. Or as Megan Pesch puts it, "This Israeli acyclovir is looking pretty hot."

She's talking about a study conducted in Israel and published in *The Lancet* that suggests CMV antiviral treatment during pregnancy may prove successful at stopping a mother infected with CMV from transmitting the virus to her fetus. The study is small—no surprise—but telling. All the women enrolled had primary cases of CMV infection during pregnancy. Forty-five of the women "blindly" received a placebo. The other forty-five took an antiviral called acyclovir during pregnancy.

In the group of women who took the placebo, 30 percent of the fetuses tested positive for CMV by amniocentesis. In the group who took the oral antiviral, twice a day during pregnancy, till around twenty weeks when the amniocentesis was performed, only 11 percent of the fetuses tested positive for CMV.

Furthermore, the study also segmented women out from the general groups and identified those who'd acquired CMV during the first trimester—when severe disabilities and death are more likely once the child is born. In the group of mothers who'd contracted a first-trimester infection and received a placebo, the virus—when untreated—crossed the placenta and transmitted to the fetus in 48 percent of the pregnancies. In the women who were treated, again only 11 percent of the fetuses tested positive for CMV when an amnio was done.

The study concluded that early treatment "might prevent termination of pregnancies or delivery of infants with congenital cytomegalovirus."

Of course, we need larger studies. We need further evidence. We need doctors to say, *We don't know* and *We need to figure this out* and to see studies like this and say, *There is hope.*

———

One of the doctors at Lutheran Hospital who's gotten wind of Lauren's and my plans to overhaul their newborn screening program is a neonatologist named Dr. Erica Wymore. Initially, through the grapevine, I hear that she's not in favor of making any changes to Lutheran's policies about CMV, believing that not enough babies will be caught and it won't be worth the cost. But unbeknownst to me, while I'm emailing Lutheran's nurses and doctors CMV testing protocols that are proving to be successful in other states, hearts are changing behind the hospital's doors. And before I know it, Dr. Wymore is not just on board with paying attention to CMV; Lauren texts me a flyer that says the doctor is hosting a dinner for a large group of pediatricians in the Denver/Boulder area to further educate them about CMV.

Let's go, Lauren texts me, underneath the invitation that neither of us has technically received.

When I email Dr. Wymore that we'd like to attend her event, she never writes back. But I notice on the flyer that Shannon Hughes, Anna's PA at Children's Hospital, is co-presenting. I email Shannon and tell her the Lutheran project was Lauren's and my baby, and we are, respectfully, going to crash the party.

The dinner is in Boulder, where Luke is from, and Lauren and I drive together, rolling north from my house over golden hills that used to be many-acred farms but have now become housing developments that almost completely connect the Denver metropolis to the outskirts of Boulder. I feel a kinship with this land and its losses, its changes. Lauren does, too. She grew up in Wheat Ridge, and she's also no stranger to loss: she delivered two of her own babies stillborn during the second trimester due to a blood condition she has, and like so many women, she found very little support in that silent, black canyon of postpartum grief.

And yet she still loves her job, delivering babies during Lutheran's night shift so she can care for her kids during the day. She loves to tell me the labor stories of her patients, and I love to hear them: one of the best is the woman who, when her baby's heart rate was dropping dangerously low in utero, told the doctor to start a C-section, right then, without general anesthetic—which he did. Currently, Lauren is making accommodations for a Deaf couple to deliver their first child at Lutheran.

When we get to the restaurant, Shannon makes her way over to us and gives me a hug. Then Lauren and I find two seats about halfway down a long table spread with white tablecloths, a fixed menu, and a flyer that reads "Congenital CMV, The Silent Virus: Updates and Controversy." I almost burst into tears, only now realizing how far things have come, if I'm reading the name of Anna's disease at a fancy dinner where physicians are filling the room. Lauren sees my reaction, hails a waitress, and says we need two big glasses of wine.

Dr. Wymore and Shannon's presentations are excellent and informative, and they impress upon the doctors in the room a real urgency to deal with CMV. But it's what happens after the presentation that I will never forget.

Shannon is still standing at the podium. Dr. Wymore is off to the left, holding another microphone. Shannon asks if anyone has any questions. A few doctors raise their hands, and Shannon and Dr. Wymore take turns answering them. Then I raise my hand.

"I'm a CMV mom," I say, and all the heads and all the energy in the room swivel toward me. "I just wanted to say thank you to everyone for being here, to tell you how much it means that you're paying attention to CMV."

Silence. Then a hand in the air. Then ten.

They're all asking me questions: When was Anna diagnosed? Did she take the antiviral? What's she like now? Does she have cochlear implants? Do we have any other children? Then from the front of the room, Dr. Wymore says my name into the microphone, and everyone looks at her looking at me.

"If there's one way medical professionals could have supported you better," she asks, "what would it be?"

I think for a moment, totally taken aback.

The doctors are all looking at me again, waiting, and I'm not sure how to condense it, how to take a world full of disabled children and their parents and answer this question adequately. I choose the place I would begin, if I could begin again, and I say: "I wish I had known about CMV during pregnancy."

But really, I tell Lauren on the way home, my answer is that Dr. Wymore's question itself is what was missing from my care.

8

———

At home that night, I think about this moment over and over again. How long I had waited for it, but not expected it. How I wish I'd said more. And I can feel that what I said didn't convey the whole of it, the takeaway for all doctors given my experience. Because it feels like medicine is missing something bigger, more universal than simply talking to women about CMV during pregnancy.

And it's then, while I'm replaying the scene, that I realize something. The problem of CMV isn't just that it's nonexistent in the narrative of pregnancy, that no one seems to know our stories. What if the whole field of medicine is largely lacking the existence of narrative itself?

———

When I look up *narratives in medicine,* I feel Kathleen's crack in the planet—only this time, it's a crack through which light shines.

In the 1990s, I read, a doctor named Rita Charon was a practicing physician at Columbia University when she read a novel that so deeply moved her—Henry James's *The Wings of the Dove*—that she marched straight back to the English department at Columbia to tack on an English Ph.D. The literary passage that so moved her was a scene between the main character, Milly Theale, who's chronically ill, and a physician, Sir Luke Strett, who's an uncommonly good listener, and it compelled Charon to become an expert in the humanities in order to improve the field of medicine.

Of the doctor's undivided attention to Milly and her suffering, Henry James writes:

So crystal clean the great empty cup of attention that he set between them on the table . . . it was like an absolute possession, a new resource altogether, something done up in the softest silk and tucked away under the arm of memory. . . . She hadn't had it when she went in, and she had it when she came out, she had it there under her cloak, but dissimulated, invisibly carried.

The crystal clean emptiness of the cup was a self-emptying of the doctor—a ridding of ego and distraction and all unnecessary noise—so that he might listen to the story of his patient, a woman utterly changed by the invisible power of his absolute attention.

Of this transcendent exchange, Dr. Charon writes, "This imaginative, active, receptive, aesthetic experience of donating the self toward the meaning-making of the other is a dramatic, daring, transformative move." And she points out, it's not just the patient who benefits from this tranquil attention; the doctor does, as well. "Do we not feel exhilarated when we can achieve this empty attention, when we can place ourselves at the disposal of the other, letting the other talk through us?" Dr. Charon writes. "Attention may be the most pivotal value in all our work—to attend gravely, silently, absorbing oceanically that with which the other says, connotes, displays, performs, and means."

The empty cup was like *hesychia*, I realize—a great, full silence; an abandonment of the senses.

It was also a form of *hesed*: the doctor's attentiveness would become a medicine-altering, world-changing contribution.

————

After reading *The Wings of the Dove,* Dr. Charon coined a term and created an entire field called "narrative medicine," whose premise is to use the critical reading of literature as training for nurses and doctors to bear more attentive witness to the suffering of others. At Columbia University, where Dr. Charon still directs the Program in Narrative Medicine, all medical students are required to take at least one of fourteen seminars on topics ranging from memoir writing to visual arts to medical journalism. Then they apply the skills they've learned through deep reading and discussion to their clinical practices. These include, according to Dr. Charon, "adopting alien perspectives, following the narrative thread of the story of another, being curious about other people's motives and experiences, and tolerating the uncertainty of stories." In doing this, the doctor and the patient enter an "attentive present" together. Trust is restored. Curiosity is lit. Empathy is stoked. And healing begins.

I'm amazed by Dr. Charon's writing. It is so poetic, so self-aware, so suffused with feeling. I want this. I want narrative medicine to be apparent in every doctor's appointment. I want this for every sick and suffering person I know—especially families facing CMV. And I'm relieved to read that the practice of narrative medicine can be implemented with very little training, according to Dr. Charon.

She explains that narrative medicine consists of three components that can be applied to any patient-doctor encounter: the first is *attention;* the second is *representation;* the third is *affiliation*. Attention is fairly self-explanatory: paying attention to the patient in her entirety. Representation is when the doctor writes down the story of the patient, in ordinary—even literary—language, and in so doing, the doctor *discovers* something they never would have known about the patient, themselves, the world.

In her essays, Dr. Charon shares the writings of doctors when they're given the creative license to transcribe the lives of their patients without computer codes, without the typical "review of symptoms." In one personal example, Dr. Charon remembers receiving a patient with a note that initially began: *Severely ill 52 yo man*. But after listening to his life story of joy, hard work, hard play, and a sudden loss of autonomy, Dr. Charon's revised note about him begins, instead: *Man of tremendous courage*.

Affiliation, finally, is the lasting connection made between the doctor and the patient—which, ideally, translates into an illuminating affiliation with all humans, and with the "fear and hope and love exposed in sickness."

———

Thinking back, the reason I feel so understood and touched by Dr. Charon's work is that I have felt the benefits of this kind of medicine—I have felt that great empty cup offered by so many providers since the beginning with Anna. I just felt it too briefly, too incompletely.

I think of Kate, the quiet and inquiring medical student in Sitka; of Dr. Vastola's conversations with Zaley about fishing and flying and all the other seeming nonsequiturs; of Dr. Kono's quiet way and his book of poetry about dying children; of Susie, his nurse, who called to check on me one summer and said, "I'll ask about Anna in a minute—but how are YOU doing?" Of the MFM who tenderly put her hand on my shoulder during my ultrasounds with Naomi in utero. I think of Allison Biever and the silence she allowed in the sound booth, waiting patiently each time, knowing that Anna might need extra time to respond. I think of all of Anna's therapists—Susie and Leslie and Tori and the ways they took Anna's tiny feet into their hands. Lori and Cathy and their thrill when Anna signed a new word. Andrew and Barbara, who shared coffee and tears and details of their own personal lives. And now I think of Dr. Wymore, who did not want a clinical report of Anna's symptoms, but wanted to look into the deep dark heart of what was missing, even if that meant acknowledging medical error in front of an audience that viewed her as the authority.

———

So what does narrative medicine look like in practice? Dr. Charon writes that when she begins with a patient, she begins with these words: "I'm going to be your doctor. I need to know a lot about your body and your health and your life. Please tell me what you think I should know about your situation." When she does this, she says, "Patients do exactly that—in extensive monologues, during which I sit on my hands. . . . I sit and pay attention to what they say and how they say it: the forms, the metaphors, the gaps and silences."

At her first appointment with a Dominican patient who has back pain, rather than asking him his "chief complaint"—a common place for doctors to start (and end)—Charon instead asks him to tell the story of his life.

"After a few minutes, he stops talking and begins to weep," Dr. Charon remembers. "I ask him why he cries. He says, 'No one has ever let me do this before.'"

This is it, this is what's been missing from my experience of CMV: someone saying, *Tell me the whole story from the beginning.*

This remedy, this form of caretaking, would have lifted so much of my sorrow. It would have changed everything.

And it turns out, the consequences of not practicing this whole-person vision of a patient and their illness are vast: "The patient might not tell the whole story, might not ask the most frightening questions, and might not feel heard," Dr. Charon warns. "The resultant diagnostic workup might be unfocused and therefore more expensive than need be, the correct diagnosis might be missed, the clinical care might be marked by noncompliance and the search for another opinion, and the therapeutic relationship might be shallow and ineffective." Meaning, the patient might give up on medicine. And the doctor might give up on the patient. Burnout happens. Bias seeps in.

Now I see: narrative is not only personal to me, critical to making visible the invisible burden of CMV.

Narrative *is* prevention.

One morning a few months after Dr. Wymore's dinner, I'm in Alaska, Luke is fishing, and the kids are chasing each other with crayons, when the phone rings. I'm standing at the kitchen counter, looking at the mountains across the water, and I consider silencing the phone because I don't know the number. But I answer.

It's the agent in New York. She wants to represent me. She thinks the CMV story needs to be heard. She's going to send it to every major publisher in the United States.

We always have an eye on the water's edge. Luke and I are sitting on a quilt, on the Magic Island beach, and Anna is dragging a long piece of driftwood behind her in the dark brown sand. Zaley is dancing with Naomi in the shallow water that hasn't yet swallowed the spit, and Luke is holding our son. Gabe was a pandemic baby, begun and born amid the fear and confusion and ruin of another microscopic virus that began with no name.

I have never found total peace with our part-lives in Alaska. But now more than ever, it's a refuge from the rest of the world. We also have a place of our own here—a small house on a rock ledge, with windows that face the same stretch of sea I searched every day the summer Anna was born. It's a view I've come to know as my own.

Anna is seven. She's in a mainstream classroom, speaks articulately, understands sign language, and sings her favorite Byzantine songs next to Luke in the choir. Once when she was six, she said a prayer that went, "Thank you, God, for giving me a great opportunity to be a human." She's different from other kids her age because of her smallness, her cochlear implants, and her subtle motor delays. And she recognizes—and often vocalizes—her differences. But being, by nature, a more logical child than a self-conscious one, she doesn't seem to mind them.

At Magic Island, she keeps turning around, driftwood in hand. She's tracing the length of her line in the sand with her eyes, amazed at the longevity she's made. More than any of our kids, she's a wanderer, lost in thought and baited by place. Whenever I realize she's moved out of sight, I'll stand up and search the horizon for her, locating her tiny frame at the opening of the forest or alongside the waves.

I walk slowly toward her, giving her space, but also making sure she's safe. She has that same mystical look she's always had, looking past the islands to somewhere I can't see. Maybe it's where the kingdom of the well meets the kingdom of the sick—a silent place, teeming with life, as shifting and invisible as the pull of the tides.

Epilogue

———

How did this book become a book?

The first agent I found did not succeed in the traditional sense; my manuscript was rejected by nearly every nonfiction editor in New York. But her initial endorsement of breaking the CMV silence was a victory that propelled me past the rejection the CMV community knows all too well. It wasn't until I found another agent—one who was much quieter in the publishing world, one whom I chose partly because her bio mentioned she was a mother—that my book sold to a major publishing house in 2021.

What does CMV change look like today?

Well, it started in 2016. Dr. Mark Schleiss, in Minnesota, was thinking about the new and improved PCR assay that had been in use for many years, which uses a much more exacting extraction and purification process to pull DNA from the bloodspot than the previous testing method, which had allowed only very limited detection of CMV. Dr. Schleiss realized no one had reconsidered how reliably CMV could be detected in the DBS now that newer, improved DNA recovery methods were in use.

In a larger-than-usual CMV study beginning with babies born in April 2016, he decided to screen thirty thousand newborn dried bloodspots for CMV with his colleague, a biochemist named Sheila Dollard at the CDC. They wanted to see if the improved dried blood spot CMV assay was actually a more viable option for newborn CMV testing than the medical world believed. They hoped they'd catch more CMV cases through the DBS than anyone might expect.

First, they tested each baby's saliva for CMV. Then they clicked out three tiny punches from the infant's DBS card to test their blood, too, for the disease. Most of the babies were negative for congenital CMV. But when the first positive came in on the saliva test, they checked the same infant's DBS, and it was positive there, too. A little while later, another saliva test was positive and so was the DBS. The third positive checked out with both tests, too. As the story unfolded over the course of the next year and a half, nearly all of the DBS results matched up with the saliva tests, and they knew they were on to something.

After two years of analysis, they considered their results. The CMV assay being used on the DBS was surprisingly more sensitive than what had been assumed: when the two labs combined their results, it was correct 85.7 percent of the time.

"This is a major new development in the field," wrote Dr. Schleiss in 2021, when the team's paper came out in *JAMA Pediatrics*. "It means that automated testing for CMV could be done . . . using existing infrastructure and requiring no new tests on the baby."

As a result, in early 2022, one year after Dr. Schleiss's discovery, the Minnesota legislature approved the first program in the United States to test every newborn in the state for CMV. This bill will hopefully pave the way for widespread universal testing of congenital CMV in the rest of the United States.

Of course, after so many years of disbelief in the power of the DBS to test for CMV, Dr. Schleiss tells me some people are still reluctant to embrace bloodspot screening as a solution. "My response," he says, "is 'don't let the perfect be the enemy of the good.' If you can help 85 percent of babies with CMV by identifying it and providing follow-up for them, then let's do it. And in ten years, we'll have something even better."

In other states, progress is varied. In California, a CMV mother named Janelle Greenlee proposed universal CMV screening, which passed unanimously in both the house and the senate, but was eventually vetoed by the governor due to its cost. Massachusetts and Indiana are also pursuing a legislative mandate to screen all newborns for CMV. And while Maine proposed universal testing that didn't pass, a bill to mandate targeted CMV testing was passed in 2022, and the

CMV task force there will gradually expand the program to include universal testing. Kathleen Muldoon is piloting a universal screening program in Arizona regardless of legislation.

In Colorado, 75% of hospitals in the state are testing newborns for congenital CMV if they are born under a certain weight, have a small head size, or fail their second hearing test. Lutheran Hospital was the first successful model in the state for this targeted testing program, which was put into effect not by legislation but by the hard work of a CMV group composed of CMV parents, nurses, audiologists, doctors, and a nonprofit called Hands & Voices for families whose children are deaf or hard of hearing.

These hospitals also provide literature on CMV to families whose babies are being tested for CMV, printed in both English and Spanish. The brochure contains pictures of Matthew, Anna, and a number of other children with CMV, and an invitation to join a local group of CMV parents.

Illinois, Iowa, Kentucky, Maine, New York, and Utah require both targeted newborn screening for congenital CMV and the education of pregnant women. Colorado, Hawaii, Idaho, Illinois, Iowa, Minnesota, Nebraska, New York, Oregon, Tennessee, Texas, and Utah require the state to educate the public and professionals about CMV—although most states report a lack of compliance in hospitals and, other than in Utah and Idaho, difficulty finding funding. And newborns who fail their hearing tests must also be screened in Connecticut, Florida, and Virginia. Ten other states have stakeholder interest in legislation. And, of course, countless other regions and cities have dedicated parents and professionals working to change the ways we educate and test for congenital CMV.

Internationally, in 2019, Ontario piloted the world's first universal CMV screening program. The same year the RANZCOG—Australia and New Zealand's equivalent of ACOG—issued a document ten years in the making that all OBs in both countries should counsel women about congenital CMV. In 2021, the Canadian version of ACOG put out a similar bulletin with objectives to raise perinatal providers' awareness of congenital CMV and educate patients about CMV prevention.

All these efforts have been led by parents whose children are disabled due to congenital CMV. The narratives of these children initiate every legislative change. And it's these intimate, personal stories that have motivated committee members in every jurisdiction to approve CMV mandates.

As Dr. Mark Schleiss says of the legislative process in Minnesota: "Compelling stories from parents is what really mattered. That this is the right thing to do is what really carried the day."

And narrative medicine?

Courses are popping up in medical schools all over America: in addition to Columbia University, medical students are learning about narrative at Temple University, the University of Colorado, Penn State, Johns Hopkins, Drexel, Rutgers, the University of Chicago, Baylor, Brigham and Women's, and many other schools.

A number of medical schools have even made the course mandatory, despite some critics' claims that listening to people's stories takes too much time and physicians are already overloaded—the same sentiment I've heard expressed when it comes to counseling women about CMV. The best doctors don't buy this. As Dr. Suzanne Koven puts it, in *Letter to a Young Female Physician*: "Often the cost of responding to the demands of patient care is relatively small compared with its rewards.

"I've come to believe," she says, "that there is no act more therapeutic than asking someone to share their story."

ACKNOWLEDGMENTS

Thank you to my incredible agent, Wendy Levinson, my CMV champion, my friend. There would be no book without the risk you took on me.

Thank you to my brilliant editor, Kris Puopolo; you gave me one of the happiest moments of my life and shepherded this project with insight and confidence from start to finish.

Thank you to my team at Doubleday and Penguin Random House, especially Carolyn Williams, Ana Espinoza, Melissa Yoon, Dan Novack, and Jaime Gordon. To my thoughtful art director, John Fontana, your work was like watching a childhood dream come true.

Thanks to the many readers of this project, at every stage: Sara Loewen, I love you and your postcards and your brain. Coralie Hunter, your vision for this project made it into what it is. Susanna Donato, you're not just a fact-checker, you're a ninja, and I'm so grateful for the attention you poured into my manuscript. Thank you, Christy and Keith Glover, for giving me the early support to believe this could be a book. To my photographer, Caitlin Blaisdell, you capture Sitka like no other. Thank you, Suzanne Gluck and Andrea Blatt, for believing in the beginning that the CMV story was worth telling.

Thank you to my Colorado CMV team, especially Jami Fries and Sara Kennedy at Hands & Voices. Thank you to the Colorado chapter of the American Academy of Pediatrics, especially Ted Maynard, Leisha Anderson, Kirsten Nelson, and Ellen Brilliant. Thank you to my Lighthouse people, whose support and smarts buoyed me through many storms: Kim O'Connor, Laurie Wagner, Jannett Matusiak, Emily Sinclair, Amanda Rea, Michael Henry, and Andrea

Dupree.

To the village of Sitka and all our friends whose stories and support didn't make it into these pages, especially Molly Blakey and Ashia Lane at Old Harbor Books. Thank you to Patti Hudson for the care packages when life was rainy and gray. Thank you to the Floyd family for being our summer family. To my neighbors Steve Lawrie and Sarah Lawrie, for all the conversations about craft and doubt and for the art studio where so much of this was written. Thank you Marica Frank, for being our safe transport to and from Alaska, my informal therapist, and a true friend.

Immense thanks to all the amazing, patient people who lovingly watched my children so I could write, specifically Kaycie Coleman, Molly Melnick, and Grace Hamilton.

Thank you to all the CMV doctors and researchers who deeply influenced these pages, even if you didn't appear on them: Mike Cannon, Mark Schleiss, Suresh Boppana, Karen Fowler, Sallie Permar, Albert Park, Soren Gantt, Fatima Kakkar, and Gail Demmler-Harrison. Extra thanks to Megan Pesch for your dedication to the way each word in this book might make people feel. Thank you, Kathleen Muldoon, for teaching me more than I can articulate about advocacy and disability. Thank you to all the other CMV heroes whose work inspired me throughout the writing of this: Kristen Spytek, Amanda Devereaux, Janelle Greenlee, Laura Sweet, Lisa Saunders, Kim Hill, and Elaine Angelo. To all the parents, nurses, and doctors I didn't mention whose work on CMV is quietly changing lives, thank you.

Thank you to Anna's therapy and medical teams, especially Bryan Kono, Susie Metzler, and Stacey Pfannenstiel at Highlands Integrative Pediatrics. Thank you to David Vastola, Susie Broderick, Joanna Stith, Leslie Girten, Lori Apley Fisk, Cathy Noble-Hornsby, Tori Hay, and Allison Biever.

Thank you to Magan and Coe Kunz, for providing me with an affordable, perfect place to write. Thank you to Lauren Ostuni for the hours of ethical and medical insight.

To David and Michael, thank you for loving my kids and me so wonderfully (even though you still don't include me in the Brother's Circle.) To Taisa, thank you for being my go-to doctor for every question, crisis, and symptom. To Willis and Anita, thank you for being my models of faith and courage. To my mom and dad, thank you for the immensity of your hearts.

To each of my children, you astonish me equally.

And thank you, Luke, my dreamboat, for believing in me, for sharing in all the sorrow and joy that went into this, for seeing things just as they are and never complaining. Thank you, most of all, for the gift of our children.

NOTES

PART I: WEEPING

000 I could not try for a vaginal birth: "What Is a Uterine Rupture," VBAC. com.

000 Once the baby's heel: Bhattacharya, "Evolution of Blood-Spot Newborn Screening."

000 Up until the late 1990s: "Early Identification of Hearing Impairment," NIH Consensus Statement.

000 But when Anna: CDC, "2015 Summary of Hearing Screening."

000 Unbeknownst to me: Russ et al., "Preface: Newborn Hearing Screening."

000 "Everyone who is born": Sontag, *Illness as Metaphor,* 3.

000 "The idea of preventive medicine": Hoffman, "False Front."

000 And less than half: Subbiah et al., "Progress in Documented Early Identification."

000 In the United States, women: "Women Don't Get to Hospital," American College of Cardiology.

000 And this glaring disparity: Gordon, "It's Long Past Time."

000 "Over half of adults": "Cytomegalovirus and Congenital Cytomegalovirus," CDC.

000 "By the age of five years": "Clinical Overview," CDC.

000 An American Academy of Pediatrics (AAP) link: Adler and Marshall, "Cytomegalovirus Infections."

000 80 percent of babies born with CMV: "Cytomegalovirus and Your Baby," March of Dimes, n.d., https://tinyurl.com/2s4w3s79.

000 In concrete numbers: Cannon and Davis, "Washing Our Hands."

000 Children disabled by congenital CMV: Thackeray, Wright, and Chipman, "Congenital Cytomegalovirus Reference Material."

000 The last thing I read: Ibid.

000 "There are many wonderful things": O'Rourke, *Long Goodbye,* 264.

000 According to the CDC: "Birth Defects," CDC.

000 Additionally, one in four: Okoro et al., "Prevalence of Disabilities."

000 "There was a level": Didion, *Year of Magical Thinking,* 31.

000 *91% of American women:* National CMV Foundation, https://www
.nationalcmv.org.

000 The first link that appears: Pereira, "Have We Overlooked."

000 "One hypothesis": Singer, "Why We Don't Care."

000 "Ultimately," Slovic concludes: Västfjäll et al.,"Compassion Fade."

000 It is true that these reinfections: Wang et al., "Attribution of Congenital
Cytomegalovirus Infection."

000 in poorer, more populated countries: Figueiredo et al.,"Frequency of
Congenital Cytomegalovirus Infections."

000 where nearly 80 percent of young: Pass et al., "Increased Frequency."

000 "I think diseases have no eyes": Cisneros, *House on Mango Street,* 70.

000 "Life is this simple": Thomas Merton, *The Merton Tapes* (1965), tape 8,
side B.

000 "Books are a sort of cultural DNA": Orlean, *Library Book,* 102.

000 CMV clearly isn't a part: "Cytomegalovirus Infections," MedlinePlus.

000 I can feel the pounding: Cannon et al., "Universal Newborn Screening."

PART II: CONTEMPLATION

000 Basically, the bulletin: ACOG, "Cytomegalovirus, Parvovirus B19."

000 "Withholding medical information": AMA, Council on Ethical and
Judicial Affairs, "AMA Code of Medical Ethics' Opinions."

000 "The doctor's desire": Rubin, "Professional Conduct and Misconduct."

000 "when, but only when": Meisel and Kuczewski, "Legal and Ethical
Myths."

000 Additionally, 75 percent or more: Price et al., "Educating Women."

000 "may represent": Revello et al., "Prevention of Primary Cytomegalovirus
Infection."

000 They didn't lose any bonding: Ibid.

000 "What I found over time": "Atul Gawande," *Harvard Magazine.*

000 Doctors disclose: Gallagher et al., "Patients' and Physicians' Attitudes."

000 More people die annually: Institute of Medicine, Committee on Quality
of Health Care in America, "Executive Summary."

000 "For a clinician": Gawande, *Being Mortal,* 4.

000 "My experience," she writes: Edwin, "Nondisclosure of Medical Errors."

000 And less than a third: CDC, "Knowledge and Practices of Obstetricians
and Gynecologists."

000 As I continue reading: Grosse, Dollard, and Ortega-Sanchez, "Economic
Assessments."

000 The last thing I read: Chen et al., "Estimated Cost-effectiveness"; Grosse, Dollard, and Ortega-Sanchez, "Economic Assessments."

000 If Anna has calcifications: Nassetta, Kimberlin, and Whitley, "Treatment of Congenital Cytomegalovirus Infections."

000 The human brain: Voytek, "Are There Really as Many Neurons."

000 On top of this: Nguyen, "Total Number of Synapses."

000 They were owl-eyed: Griffiths, *Stealth Virus*, 10.

000 He rightly saw: Ibid., 23–24.

000 "Public health saves money": "What is Public Health?" American Public Health Association.

000 I read online: Filteau and Rowland-Jones, "Cytomegalovirus Infection May Contribute."

000 "The aggregate number": Lanzieri et al., "Systematic Review."

000 Nonetheless, the numbers: Suresh Boppana to author, January 6, 2020.

000 And foreseeing: Griffiths, *Stealth Virus*, 23.

000 There could be little doubt: Weller, "Cytomegaloviruses."

000 "Perhaps no single cause": Cannon and Davis, "Washing Our Hands."

000 "A writer wishes": Hampl, *I Could Tell You Stories, 31.*

PART III: COMPANY

000 "HIPAA has impeded": Nguyen, "HIPAA: At What Cost?"

000 It's nothing any of Anna's: Dobbins, Stewart, and Demmler, "Surveillance of Congenital Cytomegalovirus Disease."

000 And Black children: Bristow, "Congenital Cytomegalovirus Mortality."

000 But it is also true: Evans et al., *Black Women and Public Health.*

000 I was impressed: "What Exactly Is CMV?" Moderna.

000 "If suffering, according to the Gospel": Gnocchi, *Pedagogy of Innocent Suffering*, 6.

000 "The pedagogy of suffering must": Ibid, 9.

000 "megaphone to rouse": Lewis, *The Problem of Pain*, 59.

000 "Almost as soon as we met": Lahiri, "Teach Yourself Italian."

000 "attended by calamitous": Bell, *Upon the Formation*, 11.

000 A few CI videos pop up: Perren, "Cochlear Implant."

000 "It is the non-deaf": Wright, *Deafness*, 5.

000 "Deafness," Wright says: Ibid., 7.

000 "We should not wait": Griffiths, *Stealth Virus*, 80.

PART IV: PLEASURE

000 Remembering that CMV: "Overview: Guillain-Barré Syndrome," Mayo

Clinic.

000 This is despite the fact: Andary, "Guillain-Barre Syndrome."

000 The Obama administration: Dennis, "Obama asks Congress for $1.9 billion to combat spread of Zika virus."

000 The Institute of Medicine has declared CMV: Bernstein,"Congenital Cytomegalovirus."

000 Namely, money is being: Capehart, "Anthony Fauci."

000 When I go to the website: "Infectious Diseases," National Institute of Allergy and Infectious Diseases.

000 enough people in Latin and South America: Grennell, "What happened to Zika?"

000 you'd need a vaccine: Griffiths, Stealth Virus, 116.

000 "In its simplest terms": Brooks, *Small Animals, 91.*

000 "unacceptable": Paul Griffiths to author, January 24, 2020.

000 And six years after: Söderberg-Nauclér, "Does Reactivation of Cytomegalovirus."

000 Kimberly Brooks agrees: Brooks, Small Animals, 96.

000 It cautioned against: Goldman, "Parenting Rules."

000 In her excellent book: Koven, *Letter to a Young Female, 255.*

000 "No," I told him: Hughes and Colley, "Preventing Congenital Toxoplasmosis."

000 Then one night: Cooley, "The One Certain Thing."

000 There's an article before me: Saint Louis, "CMV Is a Greater Threat."

000 Even if you take writers: Roy, "There's a Gender Crisis."

000 "I am a medical educator": Muldoon, "cCMV Research & Public Awareness."

000 "Significant knowledge gaps": Baer et al.,"Survey of Congenital Cytomegalovirus Knowledge."

000 Some of the most vocal: Adler et al., "Prevention of Child-to-Mother Transmission."

000 These parents are involved: "Cytomegalovirus," OSHA.

000 Lazzarroto's results: Guerra et al., "Impact of Diagnostic and Confirmatory Tests."

PART V: CARETAKING

000 These parents believe: Doucleff, *Hunt, Gather, Parent,* 179.

000 In the village: Bristow et al., "Congenital Cytomegalovirus Mortality."

000 A big reason CMV isn't on the RUSP: Advisory Committee on Heritable Disorders in Newborns and Children, *Newborn Screening,* 66.

000 using a "targeted": Fowler, "A Targeted Approach."

000 That means the newborns: Fowler et al., "Targeted Approach."

000 And studies estimate: Gantt, "Cost-effectiveness of Universal."

000 In fact, children: "Children with Disabilities and Sexual Abuse Fact Sheet," California Child Abuse Training and Technical Assistance Centers.

000 (And the Society for Maternal-Fetal Medicine): Hughes and Gyamfi-Bannerman, "Diagnosis and Antenatal Management."

000 But when the PCR assay: Boppana et al., "Dried Blood Spot Real-time Polymerase Chain."

000 Saliva and urine assays are much: Ross et al, "Detection of Congenital Cytomegalovirus Infection."

000 In a small Italian study: Gentile et al., "Prevalence of Congenital Cyto-megalovirus Infection."

000 She's talking about a study: Shahar-Nissan et al., "Valaciclovir to Prevent Vertical Transmission."

000 "This imaginative, active": Charon, "Where Does Narrative Medicine," 23–36.

000 "I'm going to be your doctor": Charon, "Narrative Medicine: Attention, Representation."

000 "The resultant diagnostic": Charon, "Narrative Medicine."

Epilogue

000 The CMV assay being used: Dollard et al., "Sensitivity of Dried Blood Spot Testing."

000 "This is a major": "U of M Study Shows Enhanced Accuracy," University of Minnesota.

000 Illinois, Iowa: "Advocacy in Action," National CMV Foundation.

000 "I've come to believe": Koven, *Letter to a Young Female*, 256.

Adler, Stuart P., and Beth Marshall. "Cytomegalovirus Infections." *Pediatrics in Review* 28, no. 3 (2007): 92–100.

Adler, Stuart P., et al. "Prevention of Child-to-Mother Transmission of Cytomegalovirus by Changing Behaviors: A Randomized Controlled Trial." *Pediatric Infectious Disease Journal*: 15, no. 3 (March 1996): 240–46.

"Advocacy in Action." National CMV Foundation, www.nationalcmv.org/about-us/advocacy.

Advisory Committee on Heritable Disorders in Newborns and Children. *Newborn Screening: Toward a Uniform Screening Panel and System*. Washington, D.C.: Health Resources and Services Administration, 2004, https://tinyurl.com/mscr9erb.

American College of Obstetricians and Gynecologists (ACOG). "Cytomegalovirus, Parvovirus B19, Varicella Zoster, and Toxoplasmosis in Pregnancy." *Practice Bulletin*, no. 151 (June 2015).

American Medical Association (AMA), Council on Ethical and Judicial Affairs. "AMA Code of Medical Ethics' Opinions on Informing Patients." *Virtual Mentor* 14, no. 7 (2012): 555–56.

Andary, Michael T. "Guillain-Barre Syndrome." *Medscape,* January 14, 2022.

"Atul Gawande: Excellence Is Recognizing Details, Failures." *Harvard Magazine,* October 25, 2012.

Baer, Hannah R., et al. "Survey of Congenital Cytomegalovirus (cCMV) Knowledge Among Medical Students." *Journal of Clinical Virology* 60, no. 3 (July 2014): 222–42.

Bell, Alexander Graham. *Upon the Formation of a Deaf Variety of the Human Race*. Washington, D.C.: National Academy of the Sciences, 1884.

Bernstein, David I. "Congenital Cytomegalovirus: A 'Now' Problem—No Really, Now." *Clinical Vaccine Immunology* 24, no. 1 (January 2017): e00491–16.

Bhattacharya, Kaustuv, Tiffany Wotton, and Veronica Wiley. "The Evolution of Blood-Spot Newborn Screening." *Translational Pediatrics* 3, no. 2

(2014): 63–70.

Boppana, Suresh B., et al. "Dried Blood Spot Real-time Polymerase Chain Reaction Assays to Screen Newborns for Congenital Cytomegalovirus Infection." *JAMA* 303, no. 14 (2010): 1375–82.

Bristow, Benjamin N., et al. "Congenital Cytomegalovirus Mortality in the United States, 1990–2006." *PLoS Neglected Tropical Diseases* 5, no. 4 (2011): e1140.

Brooks, Kimberly. *Small Animals: Parenthood in the Age of Fear.* New York: Flatiron Books, 2018.

Cannon, Michael J., and Katherine Finn Davis. "Washing Our Hands of the Congenital Cytomegalovirus Disease Epidemic." *BMC Public Health* 5 no. 70 (June 20, 2005).

Cannon, Michael J., et al. "Universal Newborn Screening for Congenital CMV Infection: What Is the Evidence of Potential Benefit?" *Reviews in Medical Virology* 24, no. 5 (2014): 291–307.

Capehart, Jonathan. "Anthony Fauci: Forced to Rob Cancer Research to Pay for Zika Vaccine Push." *Washington Post,* September 20, 2016.

Centers for Disease Control and Prevention (CDC). "Babies Born with Congenital Cytomegalovirus (CMV)." https://www.cdc.gov/cmv/congenital-infection.html. May 27, 2022.

———. "Birth Defects are Common, Costly, and Critical." https://www.cdc.gov/ncbddd/birthdefects/infographic.html. December 15, 2019.

———. "Clinical Overview." https://www.cdc.gov/cmv/clinical/overview.html. August 18, 2020.

———. "Cytomegalovirus and Congenital Cytomegalovirus." https://www.cdc.gov/cmv/index.html. August 18, 2020.

———. "Knowledge and Practices of Obstetricians and Gynecologists Regarding Cytomegalovirus Infection During Pregnancy." *Morbidity and Mortality Weekly Report* 57, no. 3 (January 25, 2008): 65–68.

———. "2015 Summary of Hearing Screening Among Total Occurrent Births." 2015 CDC EHDI Hearing Screening & Follow-up Survey (HSFS), October 2019, https://tinyurl.com/4snppj9b.

Charon, Rita. "Narrative Medicine." *JAMA* 286, no. 15 (2001): 1897–902.

———. "Narrative Medicine: Attention, Representation, Affiliation." *Narrative* 13 (October 2005): 261–70.

———. "Where Does Narrative Medicine Come From? Drives, Diseases, Attention, and the Body." In *Psychoanalysis and Narrative Medicine,* ed. Peter Rudnytsky and Rita Charon. Albany: SUNY Press, 2008.

Chen, Kai, et al. "Estimated Cost-effectiveness of Newborn Screening for Congenital Cytomegalovirus Infection in China Using a Markov Model." *JAMA Network Open* 3, no. 12 (December 1, 2020): e2023949.

"Children with Disabilities and Sexual Abuse Fact Sheet." California Child Abuse Training and Technical Assistance Centers, https://cirinc.org/catta /resources.html.

Cisneros, Sandra. *The House on Mango Street*. New York: Vintage, 1991.

Cooley, Peter. "The One Certain Thing." Poetry Foundation, 2009. Poetry-foundation.org.

"Cytomegalovirus." OSHA, https://www.osha.gov/cytomegalovirus.

"Cytomegalovirus Infections." MedlinePlus, https://tinyurl.com/yc27jr86.

"Cytomegalovirus, Parvovirus B19, Varicella Zoster, and Toxoplasmosis in Pregnancy." *Practice Bulletin* no. 151 (2015), https://tinyurl.com/4zubb9yj.

Dennis, Brady. "Obama asks Congress for $1.9 billion to combat spread of Zika virus." *The Washington Post,* February 22, 2016.

Didion, Joan. *The Year of Magical Thinking*. New York: Vintage, 2007.

Dobbins, James G., John A. Stewart, and Gail J. Demmler. "Surveillance of Congenital Cytomegalovirus Disease, 1990–1991." *Morbidity and Mortality Weekly Report: Surveillance Summaries* 41, no. 2 (April 24, 1992): 35–39.

Dollard, Sheila C., et al.. "Sensitivity of Dried Blood Spot Testing for Detection of Congenital Cytomegalovirus Infection." *JAMA Pediatrics* 175, no. 3 (2021): e205441.

Doucleff, Michaeleen. *Hunt, Gather, Parent: What Ancient Cultures Can Teach Us About the Lost Art of Raising Happy, Helpful Little Humans*. New York: Avid Reader Press/Simon & Schuster, 2021.

"Early Identification of Hearing Impairment in Infants and Young Children." NIH Consensus Statement 11, no. 1 (March 1–3, 1993): 1–24.

"Early Intervention: What Do Providers Need to Know About Congenital Cytomegalovirus (CMV)?" National CMV Foundation, https://tinyurl .com/dk9sdsz7.

Edwin, Ama Kyerewa. "Nondisclosure of Medical Errors an Egregious Violation of Ethical Principles." *Ghana Medical Journal* 43, no, 1 (March 2009): 34–39.

Evans, Stephanie Y., et al., eds. *Black Women and Public Health: Strategies to Name, Locate, and Change Systems of Power.* Albany: SUNY Press, 2022.

Figueiredo, Carla Grasso, et al. "Frequency of Congenital Cytomegalovirus Infections in Newborns in the Sao Paulo State, 2010–2018," *Revista do Instituto de Medicina Tropical de São Paulo* (August 3, 2020): e54.

Filteau, Suzanne, and Sarah Rowland-Jones. "Cytomegalovirus Infection May Contribute to Reduced Immune Function, Growth Development, and Health of HIV-Exposed, Uninfected African Children." *Frontiers in Immunology* 7, no. 257 (2016).

Fowler, Karen, et al. "A Targeted Approach for Congenital Cytomegalovirus Screening Within Newborn Hearing Screening." *Pediatrics* 139, no. 2

(February 2017): e2016–128.

Gallagher, Thomas, et al. "Patients' and Physicians' Attitudes Regarding the Disclosure of Medical Errors." *JAMA* 289, no. 8 (2003): 1001–7.

Gantt, Soren. "Cost-effectiveness of Universal and Targeted Newborn Screening for Congenital Cytomegalovirus." *JAMA Pediatrics* (December 2016).

Gawande, Atul. *Being Mortal: Medicine and What Matters in the End.* New York: Metropolitan Books/Henry Holt & Co., 2014.

Gentile, Ivan, et al. "Prevalence of Congenital Cytomegalovirus Infection Assessed Through Viral Genome Detection in Dried Blood Spots in Children with Autism Spectrum Disorders." *In Vivo* 31, no. 3 (May 2017): 467–73.

Gnocchi, Carlo. *The Pedagogy of Innocent Suffering.* N.p.: IVE Press, 2017.

Goldman, Leslie. "Parenting Rules You Can Break." *Brown Alumni Magazine,* April 12, 2020.

Gordon, Deb. "It's Long Past Time to Invest in Women's Health." *Healthy Women,* June 16, 2021.

Grennell, Amanda. "What happened to Zika?" *PBS NewsHour,* July 6, 2018.

Griffiths, Paul D. *Stealth Virus.* Self-published: CreateSpace, 2012.

Grosse, Scott D., Sheila C. Dollard, and Ismael R. Ortega-Sanchez. "Economic Assessments of the Burden of Congenital Cytomegalovirus Infection and the Cost-Effectiveness of Prevention Strategies." *Seminars in Perinatology* 45, no. 3 (April 2021): 151393.

Guerra, Brunella, et al. "Impact of Diagnostic and Confirmatory Tests and Prenatal Counseling on the Rate of Pregnancy Termination Among Women with Positive Cytomegalovirus Immunoglobulin M Antibody Titers." *American Journal of Obstetrics and Gynecology* 196, no. 3 (March 2007): 221.e1–6.

Haddad, Amy M., Regina F. Doherty, and Ruth B. Purtilo. *Health Professional and Patient Interaction.* United Kingdom: Elsevier Health Sciences, 2014.

Hampl, Patricia. *I Could Tell You Stories.* New York: W.W. Norton, 2000.

Hoffman, Nicholas von. "False Front in War on Cancer." *Chicago Tribune,* February 13, 1975.

Hughes, Brenna L., and Cynthia Gyamfi-Bannerman. "Diagnosis and Antenatal Management of Congenital Cytomegalovirus Infection." *Society for Maternal-Fetal Medicine Consult Series* no. 39 (June 2016).

Hughes, James, and Daniel G. Colley. "Preventing Congenital Toxoplasmosis." *Morbidity and Mortality Weekly Report* 49 (RR02) (March 31, 2000): 57–75.

"Infectious Diseases." National Institute of Allergy and Infectious Diseases, niaid.nih.gov.

Institute of Medicine, Committee on Quality of Health Care in America. "Executive Summary." In *To Err Is Human: Building a Safer Health System,* ed. Linda T. Kohn, Janet M. Corrigan, and Molla S. Donaldson. Washington, D.C.: National Academies Press, 2000.

Koven, Suzanne. *Letter to a Young Female Physician.* New York: W.W. Norton, 2021.

Lahiri, Jhumpa. "Teach Yourself Italian." *New Yorker.* November 29, 2015.

Lanzieri, Tatiana, et al. "Systematic Review of the Birth Prevalence of Congenital Cytomegalovirus Infection in Developing Countries." *International Journal of Infectious Disease* 22 (2014): 44–48.

Lewis, C. S. *The Problem of Pain.* London: Centenary Press, 1940.

Meisel, Alan, and Mark Kuczewski. "Legal and Ethical Myths About Informed Consent." *Archives of Internal Medicine* 156 (1996): 2521–26.

Menkedick, Sarah. *Ordinary Insanity: Fear and the Silent Crisis of Motherhood in America.* New York: Pantheon, 2020.

Muldoon, Kathleen. "cCMV Research & Public Awareness." Forum for Scholars and Publics, Duke University, October 25, 2016, https://www.youtube.com/watch?v=ALS9-rPylCo.

Nassetta, Lauren, David Kimberlin, and Richard Whitley. "Treatment of Congenital Cytomegalovirus Infections: Implications for Future Therapeutic Strategies." *Journal of Antimicrobial Chemotherapy* 63, no. 5 (2009): 862–67.

Nguyen, Kim-Lien. "HIPAA: At What Cost?" *Medical Economics,* September 9, 2019.

Nguyen, Thai. "Total Number of Synapses in the Adult Human Neocortex." *Undergraduate Journal of Mathematical Modeling: One + Two* 3, no. 1, art. 14 (2010).

Okoro, Catherine A., et al. "Prevalence of Disabilities and Health Care Access by Disability Status and Type Among Adults—United States, 2016." *Morbidity and Mortality Weekly Report* 67 (2018): 882–87.

Orlean, Susan. *The Library Book.* New York: Simon & Schuster, 2018.

O'Rourke, Meghan. *The Long Goodbye.* New York: Riverhead, 2012.

"Overview: Guillain-Barre Syndrome." Mayo Clinic, https://tinyurl.com/325tatus.

Pass, Rebecca F., et al. "Increased Frequency of Cytomegalovirus Infection in Children in Group Day Care." *Pediatrics* 74, no. 1 (1984): 121–26.

Pereira, Lenore. "Have We Overlooked Congenital Cytomegalovirus Infection as a Cause of Stillbirth?" *Journal of Infectious Diseases* 203, no. 11 (June 1, 2011): 1510–12.

Perren, Daniel. "Cochlear Implant: Simulation on Speech and Music." March 21, 2011, https://www.youtube.com/watch?v=SpKKYBkJ9Hw.

Price, Simani M., et al. "Educating Women About Congenital Cytomegalovirus: Assessment of Health Education Materials Through a Web-Based Survey." *BMC Women's Health* 14, no. 144 (2014).

Revello, Maria Grazia, et al. "Prevention of Primary Cytomegalovirus Infection in Pregnancy." *EBioMedicine* 2, no. 9 (August 6, 2015): 1205–10.

Ross, Shannon A., et al. "Detection of Congenital Cytomegalovirus Infection by Real-Time Polymerase Chain Reaction Analysis of Saliva or Urine Specimens." *Journal of Infectious Disease* 210, no. 9 (November 2014): 1415–18.

Roy, Katica. "There's a Gender Crisis in Media, and It's Threatening Our Democracy." *Fast Company,* September 10, 2019.

Rubin, Emily. "Professional Conduct and Misconduct." In *Ethical and Legal Issues in Neurology,* vol. 118 of *The Handbook for Clinical Neurology,* ser. 3., ed. James L. Bernat and H. Richard Beresford, pp. 91–105. Elsevier, 2013.

Russ, Shirley, et al. "Preface: Newborn Hearing Screening in the United States: Historical Perspective and Future Directions." *Pediatrics* 126, supp. 1 (2010): S3–S6.

Saint Louis, Catherine. "CMV Is a Greater Threat to Infants Than Zika, but Far Less Often Discussed." *New York Times,* October 24, 2016.

Shahar-Nissan, Keren, et al. "Valaciclovir to Prevent Vertical Transmission of Cytomegalovirus After Maternal Primary Infection During Pregnancy: A Randomised, Double-Blind, Placebo-Controlled Trial." *Lancet* 396, no. 10253 (September 12, 2020): 779–85. Erratum in *Lancet* 396, no. 10257 (October 10, 2020):1070. PMID: 32919517.

Singer, Thea. "Why We Don't Care About Darfur." *O: The Oprah Magazine,* September 2007.

Söderberg-Nauclér, Cecilia. "Does Reactivation of Cytomegalovirus Contribute to Severe COVID-19 Disease?" *Immunity and Ageing* 18, no. 12 (2021).

Sontag, Susan. *Illness as Metaphor.* New York: Picador, 1977.

Subbiah, Krishnaveni, et al. "Progress in Documented Early Identification and Intervention for Deaf and Hard of Hearing Infants—CDC's Hearing Screening and Follow-up Survey, United States, 2006–2016." *Journal of Early Hearing Detection and Intervention* 3, no 2 (2018): 1–7.

Thackeray, Rosemary, Allison Wright, and Katherine Chipman. "Congenital Cytomegalovirus Reference Material: A Content Analysis of Coverage and Accuracy." *Maternal and Child Health Journal* 18, no. 3 (2014): 584–91.

"U of M Study Shows Enhanced Accuracy of CMV Detection Method in Newborn Screening." (news release), University of Minnesota, February 2, 2021.

Västfjäll, Daniel, et al. "Compassion Fade: Affect and Charity Are Greatest for a Single Child in Need." *PLoS ONE* 9, no. 6 (2014): e100115.

Voytek, Bradley. "Are There Really as Many Neurons in the Human Brain as Stars in the Milky Way?" *Brain Metrics* (blog), Nature.com, May 13, 2013.

Wang, Chengbin, et al., "Attribution of Congenital Cytomegalovirus Infection to Primary Versus Non-Primary Maternal Infection," *Clinical Infectious Diseases* 2, no. 2 (January 15, 2011): e11–e13.

Weller, Thomas. "The Cytomegaloviruses: Ubiquitous Agents with Protean Clinical Manifestations." *New England Journal of Medicine* 285 (1971): 203–14.

"What Exactly Is CMV?" Moderna, Inc., www.NowIKnowCMV.com.

"What Is a Uterine Rupture and How Often Does It Occur?" VBAC.com, August 14, 2017.

"What Is Public Health?" American Public Health Association, https://www.apha.org/what-is-public-health.

"Women Don't Get to Hospital Fast Enough During Heart Attack" (news release), American College of Cardiology, March 15, 2015, https://tinyurl.com/2p8rwhbf.

Wright, David. *Deafness*. London: Penguin Press, 1969.

INDEX

< ~ ? ~ TK; please allocate 14 pages for   the index>

MEGAN NIX is a CMV mother and nonfiction writer. Her work has appeared in *The New York Times, The Washington Post, Brain, Child Magazine, The Denver Post, The Iowa Review, Fourth Genre: Explorations in Nonfiction* (where it won the Editor's Prize), and elsewhere. She was a 2021 finalist for *The Missouri Review* Editor's Prize. A graduate of the University of Alaska Anchorage Master of Fine Arts Program, Megan divides her time between Colorado and Alaska with her husband and young children.